The Psychology of the Physically Ill Patient

A Clinician's Guide

Margaret E. Backman, Ph.D.

Clinical Psychologist in Private Practice

Office of Health Services
Barnard College, Columbia University
New York, New York

and

Department of Psychiatry
New York University Medical Center
New York, New York

Plenum Press · New York and London

Library of Congress Cataloging in Publication Data

Backman, Margaret E.
  The psychology of the physically ill patient: a clinician's guide / Margaret E.
Backman.
      p.   cm.
  Includes bibliographies and index.
  ISBN 0-306-43051-7
  1. Sick—Psychology. 2. Psychotherapy. I. Title. [DNLM: 1. Attitude to Health. 2.
Disease—psychology. 3. Psychotherapy. W 85 B126p]
  R726.5.B32   1989
  616'.0019—dc19
  DNLM/DLC   88-39667
  for Library of Congress   CIP

© 1989 Plenum Press, New York
A Division of Plenum Publishing Corporation
233 Spring Street, New York, N.Y. 10013

Printed in the United States of America

To

My mother
Helen McNulty Backman

and

My father
Peter Louis Backman, M.D.

Life begins on the other side of despair.
—Jean Paul Sartre

Preface

The intent of this book is to examine the psychological and social worlds of physically ill patients—an area that particularly needs attention today, since the great advances in medical science have caused many to minimize patients' emotional concerns. However, the pendulum has begun to swing back to the interrelationship of body and mind. Quality of life is again becoming a critical consideration in treatment.

In writing the book I have drawn upon my own clinical experiences as a psychologist working with the physically ill. I have also drawn upon studies of the psychological factors in medical illness, and I was pleased to find a growing body of research. Although the book is primarily directed to psychotherapists, it will benefit anyone involved in the care of those with medical problems, such as family and friends, as well as medical professionals.

Acknowledgments

I would particularly like to thank Redjeb Jordania for his endless patience, support, and encouragement from the very beginning of this project, and for his valuable suggestions and editorial comments along the way.

Others I would like to acknowledge are Helen Stonehill, chief librarian of the ICD International Center for the Disabled; the staff of the New York University Medical Center Library; the staff of the Suicide Information and Education Centre of Calgary, Alberta, Canada; Ingrid Freidenbergs, Ph.D., for her guidance during my year as a Fellow at the NYU Cancer Rehabilitation Center; Lorraine McKune-Nicolich, Ed.D., for her encouragement to undertake the writing of this book; Molidawn Terrill for her assistance with library research; and John Backman, M.D., without whom I never would have mastered my computer.

Special gratitude is offered to Alfred Kopf, M.D., and the other physicians who participate in the Tumor and Pigmentation Conferences at the Skin and Cancer Clinic of the NYU Medical Center, where I function as a liaison–consultant, bridging the gap between patient and doctor. There I have learned how physicians struggle with the very difficult decisions they must make in a field that is not an exact science. By including psychologists on their interdisciplinary team, they reveal their recognition that social and emotional factors need to be considered in diagnosis and treatment, and also play a major role in patients' ultimate well-being.

And finally, I would like to thank all my patients, who have been the best teachers anyone could have.

Contents

III. Practical and Philosophical Considerations: The Therapist's Role

IV. Psychological Interventions: Empirical and Theoretical Approaches

Introduction

Psychotherapy: An Adjunct to Medical Treatment

To be a healthy, functioning individual requires an integration of the physical, psychological, and social well-being. Although this may seem like common sense, it is only in recent years that mental health professionals have been playing a more active role in the health care of the physically ill. These specialists include psychologists, psychiatrists, rehabilitation counselors, psychiatric social workers and psychiatric nurses (Fisher, 1986). Physicians and nurses on medical wards are also becoming more aware of, and involved in, the psychological care of their patients. Courses in health psychology are gradually becoming part of their medical training, as the interaction of the patient's emotional and physical makeup is recognized as playing an important role in recovery, often determining whether or not a person comes for treatment, or stays in treatment and follows prescriptions.

Mental health professionals can serve a liaison/consultative function, educating the medical team about the psychological state of individual patients and the steps needed to deal with specific problems. By interviewing prospective patients, the mental health professionals can identify those who may be at risk for psychological complications.

Psychological care of the physically ill is beginning to be recognized as having social and economic benefits as well. In their concern with escalating costs, health maintenance organizations (HMOs) and health insurers, including the federal government, have been looking at measures that help prevent illness and make treatment more effective. Research has shown that psychological/behavioral interventions can have an effect on disease (Schneiderman & Tapp, 1983). However, mental health providers are still only tangentially integrated into the third-party-payment system (DeLeon, Uyeda, & Welch, 1985; Tulkin & Frank, 1985). Where utilized effectively, they provide psychological support when the disease first strikes, and later help to facilitate recovery from disease; they also help to reduce the incidence of disease through educational, psychological, and behavioral interventions.

1

Tapp (1984) has described the several areas in which mental health providers have played an important role in the treatment of those with physical illness:

1. *Prevention.* This includes interventions that promote long-term habit changes and better health (such as programs in diet control, exercise, relaxation, stress management, smoking cessation, nutrition, and general health management).

2. *Outpatient care.* A large number of patients who become physically ill experience moderate to severe psychological problems. Some of these problems are directly related to the illness; others predate the illness but are exacerbated under the stress that accompanies it. In a study conducted by Maguire and Asken (1978) family physicians reported that a majority of their patients (about 55%) had some psychological problems: 22% of the patients were diagnosed as having a medical problem with psychological reactions, 24% as psychosomatic, and 9% as psychiatric. The remaining 45% were seen as having purely physical problems. These figures are probably an underestimate, since physicians are not trained to identify psychological problems and often ignore or minimize them. However, they do reflect the need for outpatient psychotherapy. Therapists can participate in the follow-up care of patients prior to or following discharge from the hospital, or in cases where no hospitalization has been involved. Therapists may be called in when an illness is first diagnosed, to help the patient through the critical adjustment phases, or later should the illness become too difficult for the patient to handle.

3. *Inpatient care.* This care includes both assessment and treatment. Assessments can consist of taking a history (medical, psychological, and social), an evaluation of the patient's current emotional status and concerns, and, if required, psychological testing. The mental health specialist works along with other staff, providing as needed individual psychotherapy to assist with coping strategies and deal with anxiety and depression, family and group therapy, presurgical counseling, biofeedback and cognitive training, stress management and relaxation techniques. During the period of inpatient care, family members and close friends are often more available to talk with the therapist than they are at other times. They can provide useful information and take part in counseling sessions.

4. *Rehabilitation.* Psychologists and other mental health specialists have for years played an important role in the rehabilitation of persons with disabilities. Their work has included psychodynamic psychotherapy, biofeedback for muscle retraining, stress management, cognitive restructuring to aid in the adaptation to loss and injury, and psychological assessment of current function and evaluation of the possible psychological issues during recovery. In more recent years, treatment of chronic illness, such as cancer, kidney, and cardiac problems, has begun to draw upon the rehabilitation model as a means of improving function—both emotionally and physically.

5. *Research.* For several decades psychologists have been active in health psychology, conducting research on the psychological aspects of physical illness and disability. They have investigated life-style behaviors thought to contribute to the disease process: smoking habits, stress, and overeating. They have looked at psychological factors related to particular illnesses—for example, the relationship between depression and cancer, or Type A behavior patterns and coronary artery disease. Other areas of research have included the effects of exercise on health, the effects of drugs on behavior, the effects of diseases and treatments on patients and their families. The social aspects of the health care system have also been an area of study—for example, the doctor–patient relationship, the role of culture in health, attitudes about health care and disease, and the effects of the health care delivery system on costs and treatment effectiveness.

The chapters that follow are designed to help those trained in psychotherapy or counseling apply psychological theory and techniques in their work with patients who have a physical illness. Although the book focuses on psychodynamic issues, working with the physically ill requires an eclectic approach, drawing upon various models of psychotherapy, including insight-oriented and behavioral-cognitive techniques, as implemented through individual, family, and group therapy. Those without extensive psychological training, such as many physicians and nurses, will find the issues discussed helpful in their understanding of patients' reactions to their illness and its treatment. The issues are discussed, in part, from the perspective of the patient, and case studies are included to illustrate how psychological issues get played out when one is sick. Some of the issues are common to many or most diseases, others are specific to a given disease. Theoretical and practical issues are discussed, and recent research is reviewed as it relates to the care of these individuals.

I

Understanding the
Physically Ill Patient

1

Psychosocial Issues and Medical Illness

1.1. THE ASSAULT ON THE EGO

Alan, a 40-year-old business executive, collapses at his desk: a severe heart attack. Six months later, including two weeks in intensive care and three weeks in the hospital, he is frightened about his health and worries if he will ever be able to return to the pressures of his job, a job that defined his life.

Sandra, a 30-year-old mother of a baby girl, has been plagued by an annoying back pain. In disbelief she heard the doctor say: Lung cancer. Now, months later, too weak even to pick up her child, she finds that her days are taken up with visits to doctors, chemotherapy, radiation therapy. She moves from place to place, unfeeling, in her own words, "like a zombie."

These are only two examples of people whose definition of themselves has been transformed: One day they were active, healthy people, and the next day, "patients." Who they are has suddenly been transformed. Priorities shift. Appointments and obligations formerly perceived as absolutely essential are now put on hold or forgotten. The ego, the central core of the self, has for the time been shattered. Their former sense of reality is out of their grasp, even foreign to them. They have been betrayed by their body; it has become a stranger, no longer dependable, dictating their limits in unknown ways.

1.2. WHY ME?

When illness strikes, particularly a serious one, the question that commonly crosses the mind is "Why me?" Some people may feel silly hearing themselves asking this stereotypical question. Yet the need to ask is there; the attempt to find a reason for everything persists. The sense of being punished, justly or unjustly, is strong.

People look for meaning when confronted with life crises, and whether in some cases they attribute their situation to internal or external factors has an effect on the course of the illness (Affleck, Tennen, Croog, & Levine, 1987; Brownlee-Duffeck *et al.*, 1987). Affleck and his colleagues, in a long-term study of 287 heart attack victims, found that those who cited benefits from the experience were less likely to have another attack, and had lower levels of morbidity eight years later. These patients assumed more personal responsibility for their lives, changing bad habits (smoking less, exercising more) and changing their life-styles (taking more vacations, living at a less hectic pace). Poorer prognosis was related to blaming others for the initial attack, and seeing outside stress as producing anxiety and worry.

1.3. STAGES OF ADAPTATION

Patients react differently to illness, which may or may not be related to the specific disabilities they suffer (Viney & Westbrook, 1981). Those working with physically ill persons need to be aware of how the illness is perceived and the meaning of the illness to the patient. Does the person feel worthless, that life is over? Or does the patient now feel special, becoming the center of attention and receiving extra care from loved ones?

People go through various stages in their attempt to adjust to a serious illness (e.g., Dilley, Shelp, & Batki, 1986; Grant & Anns, 1988). These reactions are similar to those experienced when one is faced with the possible loss of one's life or limb (Holland, 1977; Kübler-Ross, 1969: Turns & Sands, 1978). A patient in therapy once described her own initial reactions when learning of her serious illness. The three stages that Louise identified were remarkably similar to those in the literature, although she had not read in this area: denial, despair, negotiation, and acceptance.

During the medical examination, Louise was anxious but felt hopeful. Following the diagnosis, however, there was a period of shock, of disbelief, an inability to face the reality of what was happening. She felt like an outsider, looking in at the scene. Emotions were cut off, isolated from what was happening around her. There was a sense of cognitive dissonance, a temporary dissociation of the self from the body and from feelings, expressed numbly as "This can't be happening to me."

Following this initial stage, Louise entered a period that she described as despair. Here there was a conscious recognition that indeed she was involved. Feelings of anger alternating with hopelessness and deep depression affected her eating and sleeping. She was emotionally flooded with disturbing and persistent thoughts of what was to be: thoughts of self, family, friends, job, upcoming treatments, prognosis. The future appeared bleak, as if there were no way out. It was during this period that ideas about suicide began to emerge and Louise contacted the therapist for psychological help.

The next stage, negotiation, represented an attempt, feeble at first, to take control, to see if perhaps all was not as bad as first thought. Doctors were questioned regarding possible alternatives in treatment. Bargaining took place for procedures that would be less uncomfortable, with less debilitating side effects, less costly. Louise agreed to cooperate, to participate in her treatment. It was her first move toward acceptance.

During the period of acceptance, Louise intellectually and emotionally would attempt to recognize the condition and its limitations, and turn her energies to problems that she could handle. In coming to this state she needed to abandon some old ways of doing things, and to develop new skills and interests. Basically, the stage of acceptance requires a redefinition of oneself, and the experiencing of positive emotions about the new self (Burish & Bradley, 1983).

The adjustment process includes a search for meaning in the experience, and an attempt to regain mastery over the stressful event and over life in general (S. Taylor, 1983). There are various factors that affect the length of the process and the person's later adjustment (Khan, 1979): the extent of physical discomfort, the extent of limitation of physical activity, the extent of the visibility of the condition, the extent of the loss of sensory abilities (sight, hearing), the amount of acceptance or rejection experienced from significant others, and the intellectual and socioeconomic level of the patient and family, which can affect the resources available and the types of challenges the patient is encouraged to undertake.

Maladjustment is usually marked by fearfulness, inactivity, lack of outside interests, and marked dependency on the family. Paradoxically, some patients overreact by becoming overly independent, and they engage in activities that have been prohibited or entail great risk. Some, feeling that things are so bad now, may use the risk taking as passive suicide, not facing the fact that if they do have an accident they may continue to live, but in an even worse condition.

1.4. TRYING TO COPE

Coping with physical illness involves activities that preserve a person's psychological integrity, while at the same time facilitating physical recovery (Viney, 1986). Coping enables patients to keep distressing emotions within tolerable limits, to maintain their self-esteem, and to preserve interpersonal relationships. Where physical illness is concerned, patients have been found to use various coping strategies that are "action-oriented" and directed toward (1) mastering, (2) tolerating, (3) reducing, or (4) minimizing external demands and internal conflicts that exceed a person's resources (Lazarus & Launier, 1978; Streltzer, 1983).

Avoidance and denial, however, are often valuable during the initial period when emotional resources are limited (Lazarus, 1983). With certain conditions, such as paralysis, a confrontational style often stirs up anger and frustration, particularly in the early stages when avoidance mechanisms could be useful for reducing anxiety and depression (Roth & Cohen, 1986). Basically, avoidance is better than approach if the situation is not in one's control, whereas a more direct approach strategy is better if there is some possibility for control, even if only in limited areas. The implication is that a direct approach allows the patient to take advantage of opportunities if they are present. Avoiders typically delay seeking diagnostic evaluations, and thus reduce their chances for effective interventions if they do have a serious illness. Delay in seeking care has also been associated with marital problems, reports of isolation, rejection, and a sense of powerlessness (Worden & Weisman, 1975). Illnesses such as asthma, diabetes, and cancer require vigilance for proper diagnosis and treatment, and thus a more participatory copying style is preferable.

Weisman and his colleagues found good copers to be patients who have resolved problems and show little distress (Meyerowitz, Heinrich, & Schag, 1983; Weisman & Worden, 1977; Weisman, Worden, & Sobel, 1980). Cancer patients studied as part of Project Omega used a wide range of coping responses and tended to use more confrontation, redefinition of problems, and compliance with authority. Poor copers made more use of suppression, passivity, and stoic submission. Similar results have been found by other researchers (Streltzer, 1983). For example, in a study of patients with malignant melanoma, those who expected more difficulty adjusting to their illness had the longer survival rates (Rogentine *et al.*, 1979). This suggests that minimizing denial and unleashing pent-up emotions may have long-term positive results. This effect was also noted in a study of women with metastatic breast cancer; i.e., those with the greatest difficulty adjusting to their illness survived longer (Derogatis, Abeloff, & Melisaratos, 1979). Long-term survivors were more symptomatic, particularly on measures of anxiety, alienation, depression, and guilt. They also had poorer attitudes toward their physicians. Short-term survivors, in comparison, exhibited less hostility and more positive mood. In other words, behavior that physicians may consider indicative of the good patient may in the long run not be optimal for the patient's ultimate survival.

One coping strategy that has received little attention in the literature is the role of religion. Although religious belief does not appear to affect survival time or the progression of an illness, it has been found to be positively correlated with life satisfaction and lower levels of pain in cancer patients (Yates, Chalmer, St. James, Follansbee, & McKegney, 1981). Thus, for some, being religious is an important source of comfort, both physically and emotionally. Related to this is the literature on the positive effects of social support systems. Family, friends, church, and work relationships have been found to lessen the effects of daily stress, and to help the individual fight disease (Scurry & Levin, 1978–1979).

1.5. Stress: A Threat to Coping

When someone is experiencing extreme stress, there is a danger that the person's coping capacities will become overwhelmed, resulting in disturbed functioning, pain, anxiety, illness, or even death. Stress has been described as a state in which "unusual or excessive demands threaten a person's well-being or integrity" (Korchin, 1976, p. 70). It is important to remember, however, that what is stressful for one person may not be stressful for another. The psychological impact of stress is determined by the meaning of the stressor and its relevance to the needs and self-concept of the individual.

1.5.1. Stressful Situations

Korchin (1976) has identified seven classes of stressful situations. Each of these is directly related to the stress experienced during physical illness:

1. *Uncertainty and understimulation.* Stress can occur in ambiguous or vague situations, or when entering situations that are new and unknown. This describes well the experiences of those with a physical illness, particularly in the initial stages. Patients often do not understand the implications of what is happening to them. When diagnostic testing is still under way, they are suspended in a state of uncertainty and tension.

Sometimes information is purposely withheld or presented in an unclear manner, either because the treating physicians are not sure and want to appear authoritative or because they are afraid the person will become upset when faced with bad news. What they fail to realize is that the uncertainty and lack of information can raise the level of anxiety considerably. The mind begins to conjure up ideas that may be worse than what is in fact the case.

The effects of understimulation should not be minimized. Those who have been ill for some time may find themselves in a situation where there is little to occupy their minds. This can happen in hospitals as well as at home. But one should be aware that the effects of stimulus deprivation are more than just cognitive. Early research on sensory deprivation (Bexton, Heron, & Scott, 1954) demonstrated that lack of sensory input can lead to serious emotional and behavioral disorganization.

A form of sensory deprivation can occur, for example, when a patient has an operation or accident that necessitates bandaging the eyes. Tom, an

8-year-old, had been playing with some teenagers when a firecracker went off, damaging his right eye. In the hospital, he was told to lie as still as possible with both eyes bandaged so no light could penetrate. He lay there for several days in this totally unfamiliar environment, unable to see. Fear and panic at times overcame him. He listened for even the slightest sounds, to give him some sense that there were people around, and to help him get oriented.

2. *Information overload.* For optimal functioning, an individual needs input, neither too much nor too little. When going for a medical appointment, there is often a great deal of apprehension, so the state of arousal is already high. Couple this with a conscientious doctor or nurse trying to provide the patient with details about his care: information about diagnosis, prognosis, treatment. This flood of information added onto an already stressful situation is an ideal setting for information overload. The patient will not remember much of what was said. Some patients, aware of this phenomenon, take someone with them when they go for appointments.

3. *Danger.* An obvious stressful situation is one that involves a sense of danger or threat to the person's well-being. This can exist whether the threat is actual or anticipated. In the case of a serious illness, the patient may fear death, pain, disfigurement, rejection, isolation, immobility. The danger does not have to be real; it exists as a stress if the patient perceives it to be so.

4. *Ego-control failure.* This can occur when a person is forced into a passive, powerless role, and may result in depression and a diminishing of the sense of self. The lack of control over what is happening can be extremely anxiety-producing, particularly for those for whom control in their lives has been of great importance. Patients must turn over a great deal of control to their physicians and other caretakers.

5. *Ego-mastery failure.* To overcome the anxieties related to the passivity and helplessness, many persons try to master their situation, to regain control by doing something. Going to the library and reading medical journals and reports to learn about their illness is an example of trying to achieve mastery. When the desire for taking action and regaining control is thwarted, stress is felt even more intensely.

6. *Self-esteem danger.* Certain physical illnesses can be experienced as an attack on one's self-concept, and may lower patients' valuation of themselves. For example, disfigurement or severe loss of weight can affect one's body image and negatively affect feelings of self-esteem. Loss of status as defined by work or position in the family can also affect the sense of self. The ill person's perceptions may be distorted, but perception is what ultimately affects behavior and emotions.

7. *"Other" esteem danger.* Related to self-esteem danger is the patient's fear of losing the esteem of others. The fear of losing love or status can be extremely stressful. Feeling like a burden to others, or fearing that you will be rejected and abandoned, or simply tolerated, can be devastating.

1.6. Reactions to Illness

1.6.1. Anger and Rage

One of the most difficult feelings for patients to bear is the anger and rage that evolves after a serious illness has been diagnosed: anger born of frustration from the helplessness, for being singled out for this suffering, for being deprived of the life one wanted to lead. This feeling is particularly frustrating and produces much guilt, since it is hard to find anyone to blame directly. Physicians, close family, friends, and the self become targets of the anger.

1.6.2. Fear

Fear is another reaction that can be overwhelming, and may leave the person in a state of panic or complete exhaustion. Fear of the unknown, of the possible consequences of the illness haunt the patient. The mind conjures up images and thoughts that may be worse than the realities of the situation.

Fear and anxiety affect the experience of pain (Shontz, 1975). When pain is interpreted as threatening, it arouses anxiety. A reduction in anxiety can make a person feel more comfortable while not necessarily reducing physical pain. Conversely, however, the reduction of physical pain is not always followed by a reduction in psychological distress.

1.6.3. Depression

Depression has been described as the most common psychological reaction to being sick (Kathol & Petty, 1981). Medically ill persons who are very depressed and anxious tend to seek out their physicians more often than patients who are not as emotionally distressed (Tessler, Mechanic, & Dimond, 1976). However, physicians often minimize or overlook depression in patients, rating them lower on depression than patients rate themselves (Derogatis, Abeloff, & McBeth, 1976).

There have been numerous studies of depression in physically ill populations (e.g., Aneshensel, Frerichs, & Huba, 1984; Bukberg, Penman, & Holland, 1984; Evans et al., 1986; Holland et al., 1986; Rodin & Voshart, 1986). Estimates suggest that approximately one-third of medical inpatients suffer from mild or moderate symptoms of depression, and up to one-fourth may suffer from a depressive syndrome (Rodin & Voshart, 1986). Whether one becomes depressed is very much related to how severe the illness is (Viney & Westbrook, 1981), which may explain the higher incidence of depression among inpatients as compared with outpatients.

There are certain diagnostic difficulties with depression, however. For one it is not easy to determine if the symptoms are a response to the physical illness, the result of the physical illness, or part of a coexisting psychological disorder (Rodin & Voshart, 1986). Some of the symptoms of depression are not unlike those that would result from physical illness itself: anorexia, weight loss, insomnia, lethargy, and psychomotor retardation. This makes the diagnosis of depression in the physically ill more difficult. Also, patients may be reluctant to report their depressive feelings, and the depression itself may be transient and recur periodically (Rodin & Voshart, 1986).

Although there has been some suggestion that depression may be a causative factor in illness, this has yet to be determined (Aneshensel *et al.*, 1984). What can be said is that illness leads to depression, which in turn magnifies the suffering, both emotionally and physically.

2

Challenges to the Self

2.1. THE CHANGING SELF-CONCEPT

On her way to recovery after a long illness, Caroline no longer felt like the attractive, sophisticated woman she had been. "I feel like a doddering old lady," she cried woefully. "I have no energy; I feel ugly, gnarled—like one of those old women sitting on a veranda, rocking in her chair, as if life has passed me by—I can't fight anymore." Trying to regain her old self seemed like too much of an effort, and for that matter she wasn't sure that she wanted to be that person anymore.

Self-image is affected by the interaction of several factors: (a) the specific illness and the severity of its manifestations (Viney & Westbrook, 1981), (b) the side effects of treatment (e.g., medication, chemotherapy, radiation, and surgery), (c) the person's own psychological makeup, and (d) the social impact from the environment in which the person lives (e.g., home, hospital, work). All of these factors interact, impinging on one's sense of self (see Figure 1).

2.1.1. Illness and the Self-Concept

Certain illnesses by their very nature will result in their own unique problems, but the effect on self-image is not always what one would expect. In a study focusing on patients with multiple sclerosis, for example, anxieties about body image were greater in their early stage of the disease when less degeneration had actually occurred (Halligan & Reznikoff, 1985). The authors speculate that this reflects anxiety about possible future frailty and the uncontrollable nature of the disease course, as opposed to actual immediate visible physical changes. Real degeneration, which occurs later on, may threaten body integrity, but the psychological adjustment that comes with time and age counteracts the expected negative effect on body image.

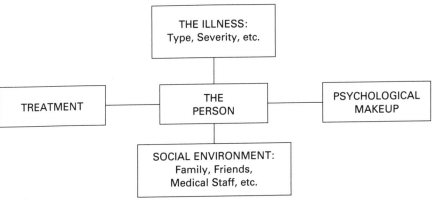

FIGURE 1. Factors affecting the self-image of the physically ill patient.

2.1.2. Treatment Effects

The treatment for a disease may itself add to the person's discomfort and be a further assault to self-image and sense of security.

2.1.2.1. Surgery

Surgery, often the treatment of choice, can significantly alter the body, but the effects on body image are not easily predictable. Healthy persons, including those in the medical profession, may incorrectly project their own discomfort about loss and disfigurement onto patients. First and foremost, most patients are glad to be alive.

Body image distortions have been noted for those who have undergone surgery for breast cancer (Derogatis, 1980; Polivy, 1977; Schain, 1982), radical surgery for gynecological cancer (Andersen & Hacker, 1983a, 1983b), and hysterectomy for benign conditions (Daly, 1976; Dennerstein, Wood, & Burrows, 1977; Roeske, 1978). In a study by Andersen and Jochimsen (1985), 82% of the women with gynecological cancer (cervix, endometrium, and ovarian) reported poorer body images, as compared with only 31% of those with breast cancer. The poorer self-image of the gynecological patient is harder to explain in light of the breast cancer patients' more obvious physical disfigurement. Although the methodology of the study has been criticized (Andersen & Jochimsen, 1987; J. Thomas, 1987), a possible explanation is that having a disease and treatment in the genital area affects the person's own perception of being a woman more severely than in other sites. Also, advances have been made in breast operations, making them more acceptable and less disfiguring. In fact, in the Andersen and Jochimsen study, the proportion of women with breast cancer who expressed a negative self-image (31%) did not differ significantly from that of a group of healthy women (38%).

This is not to say that the loss of a breast is not traumatic, or that all women will adjust smoothly. Those seen in psychotherapy may feel ugly, repulsive, mutilated, or unfeminine (Margolis, Carabell, & Goodman, 1983).Some may refuse to look at themselves in a mirror, or to undress in front of their husbands. A woman with large breasts may now feel unbalanced. No longer does she walk around nude, even when she is alone. A woman may feel mutilated, when she dares to look at the ugly scar. She may question if she is still a woman.

About one-third of the women who have a mastectomy experience lymphoedema (a swelling of the arm) within the first four years. For some this swelling is considerable, making them feel quite uncomfortable and making it difficult to find clothes that fit (Healty, cited in Burish & Lyles, 1983). This condition may make the woman become self-conscious and distressed.

The surgical procedure called ostomy or stoma can deeply affect patients' feelings about themselves (Burish & Bradley, 1983; Thomas, Madden, & Jehu, 1987a, 1987b). The procedure essentially involves the creation of an opening in the abdominal wall, to which a bag is attached to collect bodily waste. The patient has the responsibility of emptying the bag and keeping the area clean. (Note: An ileostomy is when the opening, or stoma, is made from the small intestine; a colostomy is when the stoma is made from the large intestine; and a urostomy is when a loop of ileum is used for elimination of urine.) Initially there may be shock at seeing one's body so altered. The patient may constantly be fearful of an accident, i.e., the bag slipping off or breaking, or worry about others' noticing odors. Being seen nude or being physically intimate can also be upsetting. Some patients report feeling shame, distress, and disgust. A supportive partner can be of help, but sometimes partners have their own difficulties adjusting to the operation.

2.1.2.2. Chemotherapy

The distress from chemotherapy is often more severe than the distress from having had a mastectomy (Holland & Mastrovito, 1980). Chemotherapy involves the administration of chemicals that are very toxic to rapidly growing cells, such as those in cancerous tissue. The hope is that these cells will be destroyed, or their growth arrested, before damage is done to healthy cells (Burish & Lyles, 1983). However, chemotherapy can have very severe side effects, many of which adversely affect the person's self-image and ability to conduct her life. These side effects may include extreme fatigue, loss of appetite, nausea and vomiting, diarrhea, gastrointestinal problems, temporary or permanent frigidity, loss of hair, change in skin color, anxiety, or depression. Since chemotherapy is usually administered daily over a period of weeks, these symptoms can persist throughout the series, and for three to four weeks thereafter.

2.1.2.3. Radiation

An elderly woman, who had been quite healthy all her life, had developed osteoporosis. However, before making a conclusive diagnosis, the physician ordered a bone scan to rule out cancer. As she was wheeled into the room, she felt "like a small, helpless creature" surrounded by the massive machines. Strapped to the table, she looked up into the cold eye of the huge machine. She felt all alone, scared. Afraid to die, afraid of what was going to happen to her, she began to tremble. Later, with eyes wide, she would describe the experience as terrifying.

Radiation therapy and diagnostic procedures, such as a CAT scan, can be so intimidating that they make the patient feel insignificant and very vulnerable. "The prospect of receiving an invisible treatment from a large machine in a room with no other human being present is understandably frightening" (National Cancer Institute, 1980, p. 29).

2.1.2.4. Medication

Some see the necessity for medication as a sign that they are no longer able to control their lives and their bodies, that they are now dependent upon something or someone else to keep them alive and physically comfortable. In addition, drugs can affect the patient's cognitive and emotional functioning. Sedatives, for example, make the patient very drowsy. Coupled with depression or the side effects of the illness and treatments, such medication interferes with the ability to concentrate and to work effectively, and takes much of the pleasure out of existence.

2.2. DEALING WITH LOSS

One of the horrors in being a patient are the many losses one must endure. In addition to possible physical losses, such as the loss of a limb or breast, patients endure a host of others: loss of control over daily schedules, loss of freedom to move about, loss of energy, loss of contact with family and friends, loss of identity as a healthy person, loss of privacy and dignity, loss of control over bodily functions, and, in the hospital, even loss of personal possessions and familiar surroundings.

All of these many losses, both physical and emotional, need to be worked through psychologically. This may require a lengthy period of mourning, as one would grieve the loss of a loved one (Shontz, 1975). If mourning lasts too long or seems too severe, a therapist may be called in. But mourning is natural and has positive functions: It can drain off tension and prepare the patient for later reconstruction and psychological reorganization.

2.2.1. Frustrations and Limitations

The idea of the doctor as one who takes away pleasures is illustrated by the old joke describing an interchange between doctor and patient:

"Stop drinking and smoking," the doctor orders.
"But I don't drink or smoke," the patient replies.
"No intercourse," the doctor orders.
"I'm not interested in sex," the patient replies.
"Well, what do you like?" the doctor queries, perplexed.
"Dancing," the patient says with a smile.
"Then no dancing."

Restricted activities can be very upsetting as the patient realizes that he no longer can do what he used to do. Which activities will be allowed and which will not becomes a mark of progress, as the patient looks toward being more independent. Some patients may try too hard to overcome the limitations and regain strength; others will withdraw and not try at all, falling back on old unresolved needs for dependency.

A patient who is recuperating from an illness may attempt to walk before it is prescribed, or may ask to drive a car, ski, or swim at times when others see these activities as risky given the illness or disability. The patient's own limitations and the risks involved may seem obvious to everyone around. "She must be nuts," they think. The wish to return to a former level of functioning needs to be listened to with seriousness, for it is the underlying wishes that are being expressed and which are very real. Such desires are expressions of patients' deep-seated fears of lack of mobility and of continuing to remain dependent on others, with less and less control over their own lives.

2.3. THE STRUGGLE FOR DIGNITY

The argument is often made by physicians and others that the medical concerns related to life and death come first, with psychological and quality-of-life issues a distant second. It is a strong argument, yet those working with the severely ill know how often issues of quality of life come up. Physical pain and suffering are not the only kind of suffering a patient must endure, and to ignore or minimize emotional distress may be akin to operating without anesthesia. The following example illustrates the emotional upset that can come from an attack on a patient's dignity.

Marilyn, agitated, sat facing her psychotherapist. She had just come from her radiation treatment, where her body had been painted with red lines, mapping out the boundaries for focusing the radiation. "They won't even let me wash this off. I have to go around with these marks at home, like some kind of painted freak. And today when I arrived, the technician joked and referred to me as his Picasso, as he kept adding more and more red lines to my body. I know he thought he was trying to relax me, but it's not funny. I feel humiliated and disfigured—and they stand around talking to each other, gossiping and laughing, while I lie under the machine. They forget I'm there. I'm not even a person."

2.3.1. The Place of Vanity

Changes in appearance can be considered a loss of the former self. Unfortunately, questions about appearance, such as "When can I wash my hair?" or "Can I take the brace off so I'll look nice for the wedding?" are often treated as frivolous. But they are indications that the patient is attempting to regain his or her former sense of self and to reenter the world. It is true that certain narcissistic persons may minimize the medical concerns in an attempt to maintain their ideal self-image. But if not helped, these individuals will become extremely depressed by their present poor appearance and may withdraw even more from life.

Research suggests that age affects the way physicians treat patients, and that the elderly may receive less than optimal care, since they are not offered treatments available to younger patients (Greenfield, Blanco, Elashoff, & Ganz, 1987). Also, older patients, some males, and those who do not consider themselves beautiful may not express their vanity concerns, feeling that they may be laughed at and not taken seriously. However, what is overlooked is that physical appearance is of great concern to everyone, regardless of sex or age. Some physicians do pay particular attention to the vanity needs of attractive patients, particularly women. It is assumed that unsightly scars or radical operations will interfere with their social interactions (e.g., continuing to be attractive to the opposite sex). In some cases young, attractive patients are given "preferential" treatment, which is not necessarily positive. They may be subjected to more extreme measures to achieve a more cosmetically "perfect" result—the price being high in dollars as well as physical discomfort.

2.3.2. Loss of Hair

One of the least understood or appreciated losses is the loss of hair (alopecia). This can be the result of a shaved head or body in preparation for surgery, or an unwanted side effect of chemotherapy, when not only may the hair on top of the head fall out but the eyebrows and eyelashes also may disappear.

Hair has very definite meanings to one's sense of self, and it makes a statement to the world. One mistake physicians often make is assuming that because the hair loss is only temporary, it is not of major importance.

Loss of hair is not "simply cosmetic" but may stir up deep-seated conflicts and insecurities related to the self-concept. Having the body shaved, particularly the pubic areas, leaves one bare, like a child or a baby. To see oneself like this, exposed and vulnerable, is frightening and humiliating. Although most patients do deal with hair loss, they do so in silence, lying in bed quietly accepting the indignity of it all.

Because baldness is an obvious visible statement about the illness, it can become the focus of the patients' upset. Some patients become depressed and discouraged, seeing this assault on their ego as another shameful humiliation related to their illness and treatment (Hyland, Pruyser, Novotny, & Coyne, 1984). For both men and women, the loss of hair may be disturbing because it is associated with growing old, with the loss of sexual attractiveness, and with death. Those with narcissistic personalities may become particularly upset. For some men a smooth hairless body can be very upsetting, stirring up repressed homosexual feelings. Young adults and adolescents may feel "ridiculous" and expect rejection.

Following brain surgery, a teenager complained that her face looked awful without her hair, and she could not even recognize herself in the mirror: "It took weeks to grow back. A punk haircut is not my idea of being a woman," she said, missing her long black hair. It infuriated her when others minimized the cosmetic effect of her baldness. "It would be better if they just said I looked funny or awful," she complained wearily. "My female doctor said it didn't look so bad. Would she want it?"

2.4. LOSS OF PRIVACY

Related to the loss of dignity is the loss of privacy. Medical personnel ask all kinds of personal questions, about one's sex life, emotional life, bodily functions. No area is sacred. Patients answer these same questions over and over for the scores of residents, interns, nurses, physical and occupational therapists, and mental health professionals who come their way. Sometimes patients may wonder if anyone bothers to write down what was said, or if they read the chart, or even consult with each other.

A physical exam, once in a while, can be tolerated as the patient puts his mind and feelings on hold, with both physician and patient adopting a clinical attitude. But with a chronic illness, there is the constant probing and prodding, with various persons examining parts of the body previously considered personal and private. Modesty, with all its virtues and drawbacks, plays little part in the patient's life.

The loss of privacy is particularly noticeable when patients are hospitalized. Often they share a room with other patients. For some, the company of the others is welcomed, but usually only a curtain separates them, and that is often partway open. Conversations in hushed voices are overheard, and others' tears, fears, pain, and even death intrude into each patient's space.

2.5. LOSS OF CONTROL

Imagine what it would be like to soil your pants while on a busy city street, or to be constantly, uncontrollably throwing up every morning before donning your suit and grabbing your briefcase to go to work. It is hard to maintain your image of yourself as a mature adult, able to handle your own affairs.

Helping patients maintain their dignity and gain a sense of control are important roles of a psychotherapist. Being able to discuss issues as basic as uncontrollable bowel movements and constipation bring these bothersome problems out in the open, taking away the shame and disgust.

Medical practice requires patients to be passive, compliant, and dependent. In effect, they lose control over a large part of their lives. Sick people are expected to yield to treatment demands, to be available at the convenience of medical personnel, and to regard all other life concerns as of secondary importance. When this is not possible, they find themselves in conflict with those upon whom they are dependent for care.

Some patients are wont to question physicians in detail about their illness and treatment. Often these questions are expressions of anxiety, a need to know in order to feel in control, to prepare for what is to come. Others read everything they can, to gain an understanding of the illness, to see if they have not overlooked any possible treatments. Physicians may react to this behavior as an attack on their ability, and at times an informed patient's demands may make a physician insecure and defensive.

Survival depends on patients' ability to retain some sense of positive influence over the course of their illness. Dialysis patients, for example, must endure a state of relative helplessness. Yet careful attention to the diet and the dialysis procedures can give a feeling of control and can help to ward off the sense of impotency and passivity that leads to giving up (Rodin *et al.*, 1981).

3

The Interpersonal Dimension

3.1. CHANGES IN FAMILY DYNAMICS

The increased dependency produced by chronic illness can disrupt relationships within the family (Links & Kaplan, 1980; E.A. Ziegler, 1987). Some family members may become overprotective or indulgent, fearing that the patient will die or become incapacitated. This can take the form of "anxious supervision" and nagging about what the patient can or cannot do. The patient then becomes angry and rebels against the overprotection and dependency. Family members can resent the patient's special status, thinking that no one appreciates how their own lives have changed as a result of the illness. They begin to feel neglected and unimportant in their own right, since so much attention is drawn to the patient.

3.1.1. Parent and Child Issues

Children of all ages are greatly affected if a parent becomes ill. Younger children may have difficulty working through the meaning of the illness. Older children may need to deal with issues of separation. Most children feel some sense of guilt, blaming themselves and feeling that if they had been better or more involved this wouldn't have happened.

Conflicts can surface between grown children and the ill parent. An ill parent, for example, may have been characteristically self-centered and demanding. Now, the adult children feel conflicted, being faced with the parent's obvious real needs. There is the underlying desire to help, coupled with feelings of resentment and anger at being asked to assume responsibility for someone who has neglected them emotionally all these years. They may also fear being "swallowed up" by a needy borderline or narcissistic parent, and feel guilty for wanting to pull away now that the parent is sick.

3.1.2. Huntington's Chorea: An Example

Huntington's chorea is an illness that vividly portrays many of the difficulties faced by families, where there is a chronic, debilitating disease (Tyler, Harper, Davies, & Newcome, 1983). Huntington's chorea is an organic disease, usually occurring after age 40. In the early stages, patients may be confused, upset, and depressed, particularly if they are aware of the disease's progressive nature. Later on, irritable and demanding behavior occurs, often with aggressive and dangerous consequences. The person's appearance may become slovenly and disheveled. Eventually the patient loses voluntary control over muscles, making uncontrollable "spastic movements" throughout the body. The condition is progressive, lasting for years, and death is slow and painful.

Such behavior produces severe and constant stress in the family. In addition, family members may be anxious about the possible genetic mode of inheritance and the possibility of the disease's appearing in their offspring. The children themselves can suffer from what they experience as an absence of affection, and the unpredictable, and often violent, behavior in their environment. Later in life they themselves may have emotional problems.

Spouses are caught in the middle trying to meet the demands and needs of the children as well as those of the afflicted spouse. Many divorce, particularly if they are younger; some send the children away. Others become alcoholic or have extramarital affairs, or themselves become violent, or commit suicide. However, some spouses have reported that their decision to stay with their partners occurred after they learned that the frightening behavior was related to an organic disease (Tyler *et al.*, 1983).

3.2. THE PATIENT WHO LIVES ALONE

Sheldon, Ryser, and Krant (1970) reported in an early study that adult cancer patients who were living alone had more problems coping with illness than those who had family they could rely on. This, however, is not always the case, and one needs to know the networks of the single person as well as the dynamics of those whose family members are involved.

Sometimes physicians refer a single or widowed patient for psychotherapy, making the assumption that the person has no one to turn to. Yet the therapist often discovers an intricate network of friends or an intimate that the doctor does not know about. And conversely, just because the person is married or has family does not mean that support is there. In fact, many persons who have been married have poor relationships with their spouses and children, and may need supportive referrals as much as, or more than, the single patient.

   Those who live alone have usually developed systems enabling them to be self-reliant. Yet being weak and ill can present dilemmas. Getting to appointments alone can be difficult, and the patient becomes increasingly hesitant to rely constantly on friends. Cooking and cleaning may be put off to the point that both the patient and the household begin to look run down.

   If it appears that the patient may die, problems can arise for close friends who have been taking care of the patient. Legally they may not be able to manage certain aspects of the patient's life that need attending. Relatives who previously have been unavailable now surface, out of guilt or hoping for an inheritance. They may resent the presence of the close friends and make efforts to keep them away. This can cause severe problems for the patient, who needs the emotional closeness and care of the others. Sick persons may be pleased to see their relatives after all this time yet may feel rejected, not realizing why their friends are no longer coming to visit. And tensions between the family and the close friends can create more stress for the patient.

3.3. Disruptions in Social Life

   For many healthy people there is an uneasiness in the presence of the physically ill or disabled, and an uncertainty as to how to deal with them (Bowman, 1987; Morrison & Urspring, 1987; Shapiro & Tittle, 1986; Siller, 1963). Some are unsure of what to do or say. Others are afraid of contagion, real or imagined. In becoming more aware of the patient's disability, they must face their own feelings regarding vulnerability and mortality (Livneh, 1985).

   One common complaint is that when you get sick, people stop calling or visiting. In the beginning, some friends or colleagues visit or offer their help, but gradually this tapers off. There are also times when patients exclude themselves, feeling that people will pity them or feel sorry for them. They may be self-conscious, feeling that they do not look as good as before. They may also be afraid of confiding in others about the illness for fear their intimates will pull away.

3.4. Doctors and Hospitals: The Frustrating Dilemma

3.4.1. The Doctor

   Over time, patients form relationships with both doctors and nurses, relationships that can become central themes in their psychotherapy. Physicians and nurses represent parental figures, with conflicts being stirred up related to dependency, authority, and control. They are caretakers, yet they can be cold and brusque; they help, yet they inflict pain. Termination of treatment can in itself become a dilemma.

Many patients experience feelings of separation and loss at the end of chemotherapy, for example. Not only will they miss the medical staff but they may be afraid that without the treatment they will be at the mercy of the disease again. The medical setting had become a familiar, safe haven. Knowing they may not be returning to the office or the hospital can produce a mixture of relief and loss. The many appointments had filled their lives and been a distraction; the appointments and the treatments made them feel that they were at least doing something.

3.4.2. The Hospital Experience

The role of the patient in the hospital is filled with paradox, ambivalence, and stress. In one study (French, McDowell, & Keith, 1971), one of the authors had himself admitted to a hospital for five days, under the auspices of being a real patient. He described feelings of loneliness and apprehension during his first day, and immense boredom the weekend that immediately followed. On the subsequent Monday, he was subjected to diagnostic procedures and a planning conference consisting of 12 experts—something he found very intimidating. His last day was filled with intense anxiety because he began to doubt that he would be discharged as planned. He even developed physical symptoms (i.e., pain in his legs). The day after his discharge he found it necessary to stay home from work to recover from the experience!

Theoretically, patients are the *raison d'être* of the hospital. Despite their important role, they have limited contact with higher-status professional personnel and find themselves being treated as though they were low-status persons. A study by Le Compte (cited in Shontz, 1975, p. 238) revealed that patients spend more time with aides and orderlies than they spend with nurses, physical therapists, occupational therapists, and doctors combined.

The patients also have less power to determine what is to be done to and for them than anyone else in the institution (Shontz, 1975). Being in this position can be frightening as well as frustrating, and this may explain much of the seemingly unwarranted complaining and other forms of disturbing behavior exhibited by some patients. Such behavior may be understood as an effort to regain lost power over others by asserting one's needs and demands.

Most patients understandably experience mounting anxiety as a hospital stay approaches. Therapists should make note of important dates, such as medical appointments and upcoming hospitalizations, since they may be the triggers underlying acute anxiety, disorganization, and acting-out behaviors. Those who are going into the hospital for the first time can be encouraged to read some of the books designed to help deal with the experience (e.g., Gots & Kaufman, 1981; Williams & Stensaas, 1985).

3.5. COMPLIANCE VERSUS NONCOMPLIANCE: AN INTERPERSONAL ISSUE

The results of studies indicate that only half the patients with chronic diseases follow medical directives (Haynes, Taylor, & Sackett, 1979; Rabin, Amir, Nardi, & Ovadia, 1986). The implications of these findings are immense. Noncompliance can interfere with recovery and the maintenance of life. It can also interfere with the basic trust essential to the patient–doctor relationship. There are diverse reasons for not complying with a doctor's orders:

1. *The infantilizing of patients.* The traditional medical approach, which encourages a childlike stance in patients, causes the relationship to become more like that of parent and naughty child. Some patients react by resisting on a covert level, hiding or faking test results, not taking their medications regularly, and not following dietary regimens. In essence, the patient/child is hiding things from the doctor/parent, and then is afraid of being found out and reprimanded. In this case, the physician becomes an adversary.

2. *Overprotection by families.* Family members may take too much responsibility away from patients, criticizing them for not following the doctor's orders 100% of the time. Patients react with anger, which again covertly can take the form of noncompliance to medical regimens.

3. *The presentation of a positive self-image.* Shame and guilt about their disease can contribute to noncompliance. People do not like being thought of as different. To avoid unwanted attention, patients may find themselves engaging in activities harmful to their condition, such as eating forbidden foods or drinking alcohol.

4. *Psychodynamic issues.* Resistance to medical directives can be a form of denying the seriousness of an illness. Noncompliance can also be related to fear of dependency and to its flip side, need for control. Long-standing difficulties with authority figures surface and take the form of missing appointments, not filling prescriptions, or not taking required medication. Even the term *compliance* carries with it the connotation of giving in to the authority of others. The term *adherence* has been proposed as an alternative to reflect better the healthier stance of patient self-regulation (Brownlee-Duffeck *et al.*, 1987).

5. *Beliefs and attributions.* If people feel they have some control over their illness, or if there is some predictability in its course that is dependent upon their actions, there will be more adherence to medical regimes. However, there is less incentive to follow medical advice or change maladaptive behavior if luck or fate are seen as playing a major role (Affleck *et al.*, 1987).

Treatment of diabetes mellitus, for example, requires careful regulation of diet, exercise, and often drug or insulin dosage, as well as frequent monitoring of blood or urine levels. Long-term complications, such as blindness, can result if adherence is poor. Brownlee-Duffeck and her colleagues (1987) reported that compliance was associated with the patients' perception of the severity of the condition and their perception of the benefit of adhering to the diabetic regimen. It is interesting to note that greater perceived susceptibility to complications was associated with poorer metabolic control. Perhaps being faced with disabling complications is so discouraging that patients find it extremely difficult to maintain the motivation necessary to persist with the stringent regimen.

6. *Misinformation about medication.* Some drugs, such as antibiotics, antidepressants, or anticonvulsives, may take several days or weeks to have the required effect. Not realizing this and becoming impatient, patients may stop before the needed effect is achieved. Others stop once they start feeling better, not realizing that the medication may still be needed to maintain their well-being. Or, anticipating possible adverse side effects, patients may stop taking the medication prematurely. In some cases, patients misinterpret the actual side effects of the drugs and become upset when they interpret these as indications that the illness is getting worse.

7. *The patient may be right.* Although one might assume that doctors keep up with their field, there is such a mushrooming of information today that it is not always possible to keep abreast. And patients can come across new treatment ideas, or cautions against old ones, that the physician has not encountered or considered. The patients are then left in the frustrating situation of trying to convince the physician that they, the patients, know what they are talking about. If the physician is the sort who feels that "doctor knows best," and "patients should be seen but not heard," then the patients must resort to acting out defiantly, or must comply passively with something they fear will harm them.

3.5.1. Psychological Interventions

Behavior management techniques have been found to be effective in combatting noncompliance. For example, assertiveness has been identified as an important factor in patients' compliance in the control of diabetes (Rabin *et al.*, 1986). Specifically, this refers to teaching patients how to handle criticism and initiate interactions with the medical staff. Behavioral techniques help patients learn to view criticism as constructive, and to maintain self-esteem when criticized.

Reinforcement theory has also been applied to enhance compliance. Rewarding therapeutically beneficial behaviors, while withholding reinforcement following negative behaviors, produces increased compliance with therapeutic regimes. Blackburn (1977) reported that between 20 and

50% of a selected hemodialysis population was noncompliant, depending on the measures used. Behavioral contracting and weekly telephone contracts were found to improve compliance, but only during the intervention period. As often happens with behavioral interventions, the compliant behavior tapered off after the end of the program (Cummings, Becker, Kirscht, & Levin, 1981). Wilkinson (1987) feels that dynamic psychotherapy also has a place in improving compliance, since lack of cooperation and control is often related to tension in interpersonal relationships.

4

Developmental Stages and Illness

To Linda, a young mother with renal failure, death means deserting her own baby as she had been deserted by her divorced parents. She thought she had overcome the sadness and conflicts from the past, but now as her physical condition begins to worsen, she finds herself experiencing the feelings as strongly as ever.

It is always important to understand a patient's past history, particularly as it relates to illness—her own and that of significant others. In a study of breast cancer patients, those who had observed a relative or close friend die of cancer were found to be more distressed and to view cancer as far more devastating than did those who lacked such firsthand observation (Ringler, cited in Nerenz & Leventhal, 1983). The developmental stage at which patients experience their own illness, or the illness or loss of significant others, is a crucial factor in understanding the impact of the present disease. For example, a study (Ryan & Morrow, 1986) found that girls who had developed diabetes before age 5 had poorer self-concepts than boys, whereas for later onset there was no difference between the sexes.

4.1. STAGES OF DEVELOPMENT

4.1.1. Infancy

Up to 9 months of age, children can tolerate short separations from their mother or primary caretaker fairly well (Gabriel, 1977). Psychologically this may be an optimal time for surgery or admission to a hospital; however, medical factors supercede psychological ones when making such decisions (Backman & Kopf, 1986).

The way infants experience medical treatment is not well understood, and the impact quite probably is underestimated. According to Erickson (1959), infancy is the period when the basis for trust and mistrust is laid down. At this age, there is no "vocabulary" in which to express needs. Thus, because of this lack of verbal representation, painful events, such as medical procedures or physical restraints, may not be consciously remembered later on. Because they were not able to communicate during infancy and had no outlet for their feelings, except perhaps crying, the experience remains in the unconscious. In later years these feelings may come into play again in ways that are disturbing and confusing to the patient (Korchin, 1976).

4.1.2. Preschool

After 9 months, a parent or a supportive surrogate should be included as much as possible in medical visits and hospitalizations. Fear of separation from the primary caretaker (usually the mother) peaks at about age 3 and gradually declines until age 7 or 8.

During the first two years of life, children are still very dependent upon their parents and cannot understand why the parents are not able to make pain and discomfort go away. Young children may make use of projection and may blame their parents or other significant adults for causing their disease. The initial emotional reaction is anger, often expressed as demanding and clinging behavior. If the parents do not understand the reason for this behavior and react harshly, the child may feel rejected and withdraw in despair (Khan, 1979).

Not so long ago, and still in many places today, children are separated from their parents when they are hospitalized. The separation can have a severe effect on later emotional development, resulting in separation anxiety and dependency. The children feel that the absent parents have abandoned them. Anxiety and depression set in as the little patients begin to fear that they can no longer depend upon their parents to protect them, or that they may never see their parents again.

Children may not be informed about hospitalization, only to find themselves suddenly taken away from their parents and put in a strange environment, where they may be physically restrained or stuck with needles. To stop the young patients from crying, adults may fall back on "white lies," such as telling them that they will be going home sooner than actually will be the case. This sets the stage for a distrust of authority, which can last into adulthood.

When preparing children for a visit to the doctor or hospitalization, it is best that they be told about everything that they will consciously experience, as well as the end result they may expect. Children need to be talked through a procedure to alleviate anxiety. Physicians can warn child patients about when they will be hurt: "Now you are going to feel a little pinch with this needle." Children can also be told that medicine for pain will be given during and after a procedure, if that is to be the case.

In addition to difficulties with separation, children between 1 and 3 years of age are very active and do not accept physical restraint easily. The concerns about freedom of movement usually decreases by age 7. Also, their language is not yet developed to the point that one can readily communicate with them, yet they will remember the experience.

Early childhood is the period, according to Erickson, that children struggle with issues of shame and doubt, and develop their sense of autonomy. Toilet training, which normally takes place during this stage, plays a significant role in the developmental struggle. Should the child become seriously ill, toilet training can be interfered with by the sickness, as well as by the active involvement of others besides the mother.

After age 3, children have more awareness of themselves and their environment, including more awareness of their body parts and functions. This also leaves them vulnerable to fears of physical assault, which can lead to emotional maladjustments. During these years, they also begin to communicate more coherently, but with language comes the development of fantasies. Understanding of reality is not well developed, and there may be fearful fantasies about physical mutilation for being "bad." To alleviate these fears, it is important to communicate directly to the child, explaining in simple terms what is going to happen (Gabriel, 1977; Rasmussen, 1982). Trust is important and adults should not promise anything they cannot deliver.

The interaction of psychological development and early hospital experiences is illustrated by the reactions of the following patient:

Paul, a 30-year-old accountant struggling with homosexual conflicts, was referred for psychotherapy by the surgeon who was to perform minor cosmetic surgery. Dr. W had become concerned because Paul's blood pressure climbed alarmingly while he was sitting in the waiting room. In the initial therapy sessions, Paul attempted to attribute the anxiety to events of the past week: problems at work, a fight with his sister. But he could not account for the fact that they surfaced suddenly in the waiting room. Eventually, Paul remembered that he had been reading a magazine in which there had been an article about a famous movie actor who had had a serious car accident. This triggered thoughts of blood, and then thoughts of lying on an examining table—unprotected.

Later in psychotherapy, Paul began talking about an early hospitalization when he was 6 years old. The operation was to correct a problem with his ears. It was the first time that he had ever been separated from his mother (and it was noteworthy that as an adult he was still living at home). Paul described the hospital with a shudder: very institutional, cold, unattractive, frightening. He described being frightened of the two boys whose beds flanked his. They were rough, always fighting, throwing toys over his bed. He said he had felt scared and threatened.

Paul remembered not liking the nurses. At this point there was a long pause. Then he added, "I hated the thermometer." The therapist inquired if it was rectal. Paul replied, "Yes, I felt violated, exposed." On the same theme, he said that he also hated the hospital gowns. "I felt naked underneath. Vulnerable. People could see your body. It was the same with the thermometer. I was always a very private person." Paul went on to explain that at home he still dressed by an open closet door, so he could step inside in case someone came into his room. He said he had never seen any member of his family undressed.

Paul also remembered when he was wheeled into the operating room, screaming and crying. "I felt like I would never come back. I wasn't afraid of dying," he explained. "But I didn't know where I was going, and I was afraid I would be separated from my parents, particularly my mother."

Paul's case illustrates the fears of separation from parents, as well as the feelings of vulnerability. His extreme modesty and concern about his body is typical for a child of that age; in his case, however, these feelings have stayed with him into adulthood. Children 3 to 6 years of age are beset by fantasies and often fear mutilation to their bodies. Since physicians and nurses usually do not speak directly to the children, overhearing the conversations of adults, who speak in front of them as though they were not there, adds to the terrifying fantasies, and contributes to feelings of depersonalization. When adult patients who have experienced such traumatic events as children face medical care again in life, they may become extremely anxious. Physicians may not understand the underlying cause of the patients' anxiety and may become impatient with the constant questioning, or misinterpret the patients' behavior.

4.1.3. School-Age: 7–12 years

For early school-age children, understanding is at a fairly concrete level. They tend to latch onto simple and often erroneous explanations for their illness, such as blaming it on something they ate, or having fallen into a mud puddle. With the development of the conscience or the superego, children "are inclined to blame themselves for their illness and frequently interpret illness as a punishment for being bad" (Khan, 1979). The child's emotional reactions typically fluctuate between being angry at significant others, such as parents or doctors, and blaming themselves.

As they get older, their understanding of reality develops more fully, and they tend to deal with anxiety through intellectualization (Erickson, 1959). During this period, the child has need for information that is clear, relevant, and realistic. Concrete explanations begin to give way to more valid understandings of the cause of the illness. When working as a liaison/consultant to physicians, therapists can suggest that the physician take time to talk to the child and to make an ally of the child. If surgery or hospitalization is required, a brief rundown of what to expect is suggested, including, if possible, a visit to the site.

During these early school years, children may tolerate the effects of illness better than when older or younger (Gabriel, 1977). Although they still need adequate support and preparation, they can tolerate separation from parents better than younger children, and are less involved in the turmoil of adolescence. They can make use of intellectualization and rationalization, and their anxieties can be lessened by clear explanations of what is about to happen.

4.1.4. Puberty and Adolescence

By the beginning of puberty, a child's emotional reactions become more complex. The question "Why me?" begins to be heard. Such children may feel sorry for themselves and brood for days. Philosophic and religious explanations may be used to help children deal with the illness.

The struggle for identity marks adolescence, and group acceptance and recognition becomes important (Erickson, 1959). When adolescents become ill, feelings of inadequacy and of not being a complete person can dominate their thoughts. Self-esteem, which is shaped by peer reinforcement, can suffer. Some teens carry denial to an extreme and act in ways that are actually detrimental to their health, i.e., drinking alcohol when contraindicated by medication, or engaging in strenuous sports after the diagnosis of a congenital heart problem. This pattern can continue throughout life.

Although the cosmetic implications of an illness are important at all ages, they are of considerable significance in adolescence, when appearance, identity, and acceptance become of prime concern. Facial disfigurement or physical disabilities may affect self-image. Drugs, such as steroids, may alter physical appearance (e.g., shorten stature), which can be of great concern, particularly to males. How these problems are handled depends in large part upon the reactions of others.

Adolescents worry about loss of control. When a serious illness develops later in life, there may be a certain amount of regression. The young person may become more dependent on, and demanding of, peers and friends, or may withdraw and be sad for many months. There may be problems with schoolwork, social relations, and personal habits. Periodic illness may cause the young person to miss school and may affect academic performance and socialization. Physical activity and athletic participation may be restricted, isolating the patient from peers. The young patient may be ostracized and discriminated against in many obvious or subtle ways (Stoudemire, 1985).

A chronic illness may foster dependency on others and lead to various kinds of rebellious angry acting-out, as a reaction to the limitations and the dependency (Stoudemire, 1985). Patients who have diabetes from childhood, for example, may have intense unresolved dependency needs (Boehnert & Popkin, 1986). They may never have fully passed through the stages of separation and individuation, or achieved the sense of independence normally reached by the end of adolescence. Parents may have been, and still may be, overinvolved and infantilizing. As adults, these individuals will probably have difficulty functioning independently in work, studies, and other aspects of their daily life.

4.2. ANESTHESIA: EFFECTS ON EMOTIONAL AND COGNITIVE DEVELOPMENT

Although medical concerns always supercede the psychological in making decisions regarding treatment, the long-term effects of the medical interventions on the person's later development are often not known, or are minimized. Anesthesia is a point in fact. Some operations do not need to be performed immediately, and the question arises about the optimal time to operate given the child's social and psychological stage of development. In addition to issues such as separation, level of comprehension, and body integrity, the effect of general anesthesia needs to be taken into account. However, little is known about the effects of anesthesia on a child's later cognitive or emotional development (Backman & Kopf, 1986). Some research with mice *in utero* have shown learning deficits in later generations (Chalon *et al.*, 1981, 1983). However, no long-term studies with humans have been conducted. Anesthesiologists usually prefer not to give general anesthesia before 9 to 12 months of age, because the child's respiratory and circulatory systems are not yet fully developed until that time.

Psychoanalytic practitioners have suggested, however, that earlier experiences with anesthesia may leave their mark on the psyche (Weinberger & Kantor, 1976–1977). Those who had general anesthesia before age 3 may now, as adults, under certain stressful conditions, experience isolated symptoms that mimic other types of psychosomatic reactions: shortness of breath, tics, feelings of unreality, a floating sensation, numbness around the mouth, gagging, coughing, gastric discomfort, and various bodily pains.

Those who had general anesthesia after age 3, when verbal and cognitive functions were more mature, may exhibit more complex neurotic patterns as they grow older, rather than isolated symptoms. The original trauma may interact with unresolved issues in the person's developmental stage, only to reappear later as fear of physical mutilation, or fear of abandonment, submission, and helplessness.

Having to undergo anesthesia, specifically general anesthesia, can be upsetting for many patients, children and adults, and a great deal of trust is given to the anesthesiologist (J.M. Garfield, 1974). Loss of control and fears of death are issues that come to the fore. Those who were given anesthesia via a mask may have feelings of suffocation when anticipating upcoming surgery, or in other stressful situations. Early childhood experiences may surface—for example, remembering when your sister put a pillow over your head. Although patients may eventually be able to discuss their anxieties with a therapist, they may be reluctant to bring them to the attention of the physician, feeling they will not be taken seriously.

4.3. THE CHILD'S REACTION TO ILLNESS IN THE FAMILY

The developmental stage also needs to be taken into account when a patient has lived through the illness and possible death of a significant other. Therapists should make special note of the age at which these events occurred. Although parents may try to hide their own suffering, children sense what is going on. If not allowed to verbalize their fears and feelings, then they become internalized, only to resurface later in maladaptive emotional responses. Issues of separation can arise, as well as feelings of being punished for being bad. "My mother has become ill, or was taken away, because of me." Another's illness can also cause great anxiety in the child who fears having the same illness; again, fantasies and fears of mutilation and vulnerability come to the fore.

The illness of siblings can be particularly intense. If an older sibling becomes chronically ill, younger siblings may suffer adjustment problems, partly because they feel to blame and partly because they feel they are not getting the attention they need. They may also see that being sick has its rewards. And resentment toward the sick brother or sister may persist throughout adulthood.

4.4. PARENTAL REACTIONS TO A CHILD'S ILLNESS

Following the diagnosis of a child's serious illness, parents may react with acute anxiety and fear. Later this may turn to denial and disbelief, particularly if the child does not outwardly appear to be very sick. Guilt, shame, and mourning may follow, depending upon the circumstances of the disease. The search for the cause of the illness can arouse all sorts of fantasies and explanations related to heredity, pregnancy, child care, and even religious beliefs. If the parents feel that one of them passed it on to the child, guilt may follow, leading to overprotectiveness. Parents scrutinize all aspects of their child's early life for possible neglect, abuse, or misjudgment on their part or on the part of others. In one case, the parents of a baby who was born with a large red growth on his face blamed this congenital deformity on a meal of spicy Mexican food the mother had craved and consumed during pregnancy. In another case, political refugees blamed their infant's congenital abnormality on the stress they experienced during their period in exile. This caused them to feel much guilt for having put their own needs first and jeopardizing their child's health.

It is not uncommon for marriages to break up because one becomes overly involved with the sick child and the other is hardly involved at all (Khan, 1979). Well-adjusted parents do not excessively sympathize or over-protect a sick child; instead, they try to help such children develop their full potential in social and educational areas.

II
Treating the Physically Ill Patient

5

Psychodynamic Issues

5.1. DEFENSE MECHANISMS

The distinction is often made between coping and defense mechanisms. Both are protective of the individual, and both provide some satisfaction for needs. Coping responses, however, are flexible and adaptive. They are more under conscious control and are considered more effective. Defenses, on the other hand, are more rigid patterns of behavior that ultimately may be maladaptive, and they usually operate automatically without conscious awareness. They allow the person to continue functioning, although in a more limited and inflexible way.

Each physically ill person brings to the situation his or her own unique constellation of defenses. Under the stress of the illness, however, the defenses may begin to break down, leaving the person overwhelmed and unable to cope with the illness, or with everyday matters and concerns. In some cases, defenses that were typical of the person's premorbid personality—for example, avoidance or denial—may become even more rigid as a way of helping the person deal with the enormity of the present situation. Although experienced therapists may be quite familiar with these psychological defenses, it is important to note how they get played out when a patient is under the stress of a severe illness.

5.1.1. Repression

Repression is the blocking from consciousness of troubling ideas and emotions. They may be current feelings or happenings, or memories and fears from childhood that have remained unexpressed and distorted in the unconscious. When a person becomes ill, or has been ill for some time, the repressed feelings (e.g., issues of dependency and abandonment) may rise to the surface in an overwhelming way.

If there is a recurrence of a previous illness, the fact that the patient has gone through this before is no reason to assume that it will be easier this time. Familiarity does not necessarily breed understanding and acceptance. Upon recurrence, the person is thrown into the adjustment process once again in facing the possibility of pain, disfigurement, or immobility, the discomfort of treatment, and the threat of death (Holland, 1977). Many patients find it more difficult the second time around, reporting feeling even more desolate than before, the hope of cure gone (Koocher, 1986; Koocher & O'Malley, 1981). Also, having to relive the experience, an experience one thought had been put to rest, reawakens anxieties and conflicts that for long the person may have been able to ignore. As one patient exclaimed: "I thought I had all this behind me; I don't know if I can go through it again."

Ann's left leg had been amputated when she was 17 because of a malignant tumor. Now a happily married woman of 35, with two children and a good job, she is told by a surgeon that she has a cancerous tumor of the breast. The surgeon recommends a mastectomy immediately—"reassuring her" that "this will be nothing," since she has already lost a leg. Ann's outrage at the physician's insensitivity was delayed until she reached home, where following the initial shock she broke down, overcome with anger and despair. Not only did the physician fail to recognize the intense emotional reactions patients have to illness, but he minimized to the point of distortion the meaning of the past experience in the present situation. Subsequently, Ann changed surgeons and had a small benign tumor removed from her breast.

When an illness reappears or when treatment is extended over time, physicians may feel a sense of failure, and may themselves attempt to deny the patient's despair. They may assume that familiarity with the illness and treatment gives the patient understanding and strength. In fact, it may awaken old fears, as well as creating new ones. Facing the third in a series of operations, for example, may be more anxiety-producing than the earlier ones. "Now I know what to worry about," a patient confesses. Or, "I was lucky the first two times. Maybe my luck is running out. After all, how many times can you go through this without a problem?"

In a review of the research, Beutler, Engle, Oro'-Beutler, Daldrup, and Meredith (1986) concluded that prolonged blocking or inhibition of intense interpersonal anger may be a common correlate of depression, chronic pain, and susceptibility to disease. They also concluded that blocked and suppressed emotional experience that coincides with prolonged stress may also result in deactivation of the body's production of natural killer cells, which are associated with the ability to ward off disease, pain, and depression (p. 756). This lends support to the notion that discussing emotionally laden traumatic events can have a positive effect on one's physical health. However, the effect is greatest if the negative emotions are directed against whatever is experienced as blocking the action. The patients need to feel that their expression of anger or other emotions will have some positive effect. If the emotional release continues to be directed toward a goal that cannot be fulfilled, little therapeutic benefit can be expected.

5.1.2. Denial and Avoidance

Denial, the psychological inability to accept what has occurred, is a very common defense where physical illness and disability are concerned. Although intellectually a person may know what has happened, the seriousness or the implications are ignored or minimized. Denial may show itself as numbness, removal of material from consciousness, and avoidance of reminders of the condition. It can take the form of consciously or unconsciously refusing to accept the limitations imposed upon one: A cardiac patient begins to smoke heavily again; a person, not long after a series of delicate orthopedic operations, undertakes strenuous risk-taking exercises and activities. The need to get some relief from an extended illness and its treatment can lead patients to deny or underreact when something is genuinely wrong. With diabetic patients, for example, problems with vision might be ignored, until the patient is confronted with the realities of the deteriorating condition or is totally unable to function. In such cases, denial does not serve a protective function but creates even more complications in the long run.

The results of a longitudinal study of patients with coronary heart disease suggests that denial is helpful in a limited time frame, during the acute phase of a critical illness, but can extract a price later on (Levine *et al.*, 1987). When compared with "low deniers," "high deniers" spent fewer days in intensive care and had fewer signs of cardiac dysfunction during their hospitalization. However, during the year following discharge, the high deniers did not adapt as well, showed less compliance with medical recommendations, and required more days of further hospitalization.

When faced with denial, a therapist must make decisions about how much to help the patient confront the reality of the situation. If family and professionals go along with denial, patients can become fearful that they are at fault for having the symptoms, or are in fact too fragile to deal with the realities of their condition. A lack of direct discussion for fear of upsetting patients only reinforces the denial, making it more difficult for them to come to terms with their condition. On the other hand, when confronted with frightening issues, a patient may begin to look for another physician or therapist, considering such discussion evidence of "negative thinking" (Boehnert & Popkin, 1986).

Another negative effect is that denial, over the long term, may interfere with the protective function of the immunological system. In one study (Levy, Herberman, Maluish, Schlien, & Lippman, 1985), women with breast cancer who appeared to have accepted their diagnosis and denied emotional distress had lower natural killer cell counts and were more likely to die of breast cancer than those who readily admitted to emotional and psychological distress. If this result is generally so, then it is another refutation of the argument that psychotherapy is too upsetting for patients. Getting them to talk about their emotional distress, rather than bottling it up and acting like "good patients," is apparently related to better physical and mental health.

5.1.3. Isolation of Affect

Isolation of affect is a partial repression of emotions, a splitting off of thoughts from feelings. It may take the form of patients' blandly discussing their illness and its impact on themselves or the family. This behavior can be mistaken for good adjustment. Busy professionals may prefer such behavior in a patient, since the unemotional patient is easier to deal with. But as stress continues, the isolation of affect may not be sufficient to keep the underlying anxieties and rage in check. Not having worked through the issues involved, the patient may at some point dissemble.

A healthier version of isolation of affect is when a patient dissociates a diseased part of the body from the self. Someone who has had a breast removed may speak of the absent breast with clinical distance, while recognizing that somehow this adjustment is odd: "I saw it as something diseased that was no longer a part of my body, and I had to get rid of it. I'm talking as thought it wasn't part of me."

5.1.4. Intellectualization

Intellectualization is another way of separating feelings from thoughts. With this defense there is an emphasis on logic and knowledge. It is an attempt to try to take control in a situation where one feels vulnerable and out of control. Intellectualization can take the form of reading about one's illness and asking questions in an attempt to understand the nature and course of the disease.

5.1.5. Regression

Under the impact of a serious illness, a person's behavior may regress to that of an earlier period—for example, crying, becoming helpless and dependent. When the patient feels overwhelmed and unable to cope, adopting childlike behavior may make others step in to take charge and to comfort. This can be seen as a way of satisfying present needs, while defending against further distress and disorganization. If the regressive behavior continues for long, it may cause strains between the patient and family members or other caretakers, who begin to tire of the constant demand for attention and the person's not fulfilling usual duties.

5.1.6. Resistance

Chronically ill patients may be "overdoctored" and thus resistant to spending the additional time or money to see a psychotherapist. They may have been using a great deal of denial in dealing with their illness, and continue to use it when faced with their emotional problems. As a result of the overwhelming anxiety related to the illness, they may be quite reluctant to enter psychotherapy. "I need all the emotional strength I can muster, just to get through each day. I don't know if I can handle it, if it opens up any more doors." They may also interpret going to a psychotherapist as admitting that they have lost control over their illness and their life.

Resistance to treatment is also a concern to the medical staff. Not taking prescription drugs, not following medical advice, missing appointments, argumentative behavior can all be symptomatic of resistance. It is easy for the physician or nurse to become angered at the patient who seems uncooperative, but understanding that these behaviors are part of the patients' armor against anxiety and lack of control over their bodies will put this frustrating behavior into perspective. Sometimes resistance, like its counterparts, negativism and regression, can also be a way of drawing attention to oneself, a cry for help.

5.2. Transference

Theoretically, transference is the tendency to displace onto another person emotions originally felt toward parents or other significant persons in one's past (Menninger, 1958). If repressed needs and memories from earlier experiences have not been worked through, the new relationship may be misjudged, incorrectly evaluated, or distorted in some way.

5.2.1. Transference and the Psychotherapist

One of the roles of a psychotherapist is to help patients, through the therapeutic process, to gain an understanding of how their feelings and actions affect and are affected by others. Relationships with others are particularly important when a person becomes physically ill, because the very nature of the interpersonal relationships changes as a result of illness. An independent person may become more dependent on friends, spouse, children, or professionals, including doctors, nurses, and the psychotherapist. Conflicts arise over the need to be taken care of, and the desire for independence and sense of self. Before the illness a certain adjustment or balance may have been established, but now the structure has been shaken and unresolved issues resurface: Who has power? Who makes demands? Who is the center of attention?

Once the initial resistance to psychotherapy is worked through, the patient may quickly become dependent on the therapist, needing someone to understand, to listen, and, in some "unknown" way, to help. It is not uncommon for the therapist to be experienced as filling the needs of a mother, one who is there for you when you are sick. These transference feelings can arise much more quickly and more strongly in therapy with the physically ill because the patient is in crisis, which breaks down many of the defenses. Anger, idealization, and dependency are only a few of the transference signs that signal the existence of a transference relationship. Working through resistance is a way of beginning to understand the transference feelings that stand in the way of forming mature relationships, something that becomes of primary importance when illness requires a shift in roles and brings new people into the patient's life space.

5.2.2. Transference and the Medical Staff

The patients' special relationship to their physicians and the medical establishment triggers conflicts revolving around issues of dependency and relationships to authority figures. The physician who spends time with the patient, who gets to know the patient personally, may be experienced as warm and caring. A more aloof, distant, evasive attitude, common to many busy specialists, may anger patients, particularly those who have unresolved needs from emotionally unavailable or critical parents.

When a physician refers a patient for psychotherapy, transference feelings, usually negative at first, are operating. The purpose of the referral may be misunderstood by the patient, who has placed great faith in "my doctor." For one, the referral may shake confidence in the physician, who is admitting there are areas he or she cannot handle. The referral can also be experienced as abandonment by the physician who is no longer able to treat or be interested in the patient.

Bob adores his physician, Dr. A, whom he sees as the caring father he never had. He feels comfortable confiding in Dr. A, who seems interested in him personally as well as medically. Dr. A realizes after a while that Bob has some deep psychological problems, but when he tries to refer Bob for psychological help, Bob refuses. He feels confused and frightened. Can this mean that Dr. A no longer cares for him? Does he no longer want to spend time talking to him? Can he no longer treat him? Feelings of rejection and disappointment set in. Bob eventually agrees to give therapy a try, after Dr. A reassures him that the psychotherapy referral is part of the regular procedures, which involve a team approach intended to support patients emotionally through the rough times.

5.3. COUNTERTRANSFERENCE

The carry-over of feelings into a new relationship is bidirectional, with both parties bringing to the interaction their own needs and expectations. Just as *transference* is the term applied to the patient's carry-over into the present situation, *countertransference* refers to the professional's emotional reactions to the patient (Fromm-Reichmann, 1950; Menninger, 1958; Sullivan, 1947). Positive feelings and empathy toward a patient can be very helpful. But there are pitfalls to watch out for when either positive or negative feelings come into play.

5.3.1. Countertransference and the Medical Staff

Countertransference affects the way a physician or nurse treats patients—the extent to which he or she moves toward or away from them. A woman patient who reminds the physician of his first love may get extra attention, whereas the older woman, who cries and moans in his office, may remind him of his nagging, hypochondriacal mother. He reacts by assuming a very rushed and busy manner, keeping contact to a minimum. Yet the physician may be unaware that he is acting differently toward these patients.

Physicians and nurses may find themselves referring patients for psychotherapy out of hostility, possibly for noncompliance with treatment, or because of their own inability to deal with the patients' tears and despondency. These may in actuality be valid circumstances for making a referral; however, the professionals should be aware of their own countertransference feelings, so that in making the referral they do so with the same professional authority that they would a medical referral. Otherwise, the patients, who are often very perceptive, will sense that something is not right and feel rejected, and rightfully so.

Anger, anxiety, feelings of helplessness, and even sexual arousal are cues that countertransference may be operating. Being aware of these feelings toward patients helps the professionals maintain control over their behavior and over the situation. Young students in training should be particularly aware of their countertransference feelings, so that in the formation of their professional manner they do not acquire defenses or ways of responding that are counterproductive.

5.3.2. Countertransference and the Psychotherapist

When a therapist's private patient becomes ill, practical problems, as well as countertransference feelings, arise. The therapist may initially join with the patient in denying the significance of the physical symptoms, such as extreme tiredness, irritability, and aches and pains. The therapist may fear the loss of the relationship or the loss of money, should the patient be seriously ill. Or the therapist may feel guilty, wondering if he or she should have done more, by acting earlier or encouraging the patient more strongly to seek help.

In addition to the usual countertransference issues that arise in psychotherapy, therapists need to be specifically aware of their feelings when working with those who are physically ill, disabled, or disfigured—for example, fear of contagion, revulsion at an unsightly wound or deformity, disgust at intimate talk about the details of operations or bowel movements. As part of psychotherapy training therapists learn not only to be aware of countertransference feelings but to control their reactions, both verbal and nonverbal. Body language speaks as much as words. Patients become hyperviligant and scrutinize facial expressions for the slightest signs of discomfort. A pulling back or a sudden twist in the chair at the mention of something unpleasant may be interpreted as rejection or fear on the therapist's part. Although at one time or another most therapists may have a negative reaction to what they see or hear, with training and experience they become attuned to these feelings. They do not pretend that everything is all right, but they learn to show empathy and understanding. They also learn to use their own reactions to help them understand how others might react to the patient, providing insight into how the illness affects the patient's self-concept and interpersonal relations.

Beginning therapists are often unprepared for what is to come, and they feel a sense of helplessness since they are unable to cure the disease. If the therapist feels insecure and hesitant, these feelings get communicated to the patient. A close working relationship with the physician involved in the care of the patient is useful for overcoming many of the negative countertransference feelings. Understanding the cause and course of the disease helps the therapist know which of the patient's behaviors and ideas to support, and also prepares the therapist for what is to come. One of the best ways to overcome negative transference feelings is to focus not solely on the disease but on the patient as a person who happens to have an illness as one of many of life's occurrences.

Sometimes people enter the mental health professions or begin working with those with a physical illness because they or someone close to them has had similar problems. Drawing upon one's personal experience can have its limitations, however, since one may expect the patient's reactions and experiences to mirror one's own. This is seldom the case. The therapist needs to be open to hearing what the patient is actually saying and feeling. When and if to share is a very delicate question. Knowing that the therapist has, or has had, the same illness may be reassuring to some patients; on the other hand, it may cause others to become overly concerned about the health of the therapist, or worried that the therapist is more concerned with his own problems—that theirs are not as important. It is always of ultimate importance for the therapist to understand the reasons and the underlying countertransference issues when sharing reactions or personal data with patients. Is the therapist looking for sympathy? Trying to show how courageous she is? Looking for power? Trying to reassure herself? Competing with the patient?

6
Personality and Physical Illness

6.1. PERSONALITY STYLE AND ADAPTATION TO ILLNESS

Depending upon their personalities, patients find different aspects of their illnesses upsetting and use different techniques for coping with these difficulties (Geringer & Stern, 1986):

6.1.1. Borderline

Patients with borderline characteristics present some of the most difficult problems in patient management. They typically are impulsive and unpredictable, are very manipulative, and can alternate between idealizing someone (e.g., the physician) at one time and devaluing him or her at another. At times they appear normal; however, their mood can shift quite markedly to depression, anxiety, or irritability, and they are capable of intense, and often inappropriate rage.

Illness is experienced by those with borderline personality characteristics as a conflict between the wish for boundless care and the threat of abandonment. Despite a demand for direction and support, borderline patients have been known to consistently and deliberately refuse to follow medical advice. They enter treatment with their own agendas, including the desire to be rescued, a hope for a magical cure, and fantasies of being fought over by the treating professionals.

During psychotherapy, there may be suicide attempts, numerous emergency room visits, and efforts to split the staff. Their behavior produces feelings of anger and frustration in the professionals who try to help them. Initial sessions are marked by denial, depression, extreme dependency, enraged outbursts, and resistance to dealing with substantive issues involved in their care. Such patients are very demanding and often express anger at the physician or therapist for not being always available. They respond best to gentle but firm limit-setting, particularly on the amount of time spent with them. Therapy can be expected to be long-term and difficult, with frequent regression, primitive thinking, and possible decompensation into psychosis (Boehnert & Popkin, 1986). It may take up to a year to form a therapeutic alliance, which is necessary before real work involving the physical disease can begin.

6.1.2. Obsessive–Compulsive

Those with compulsive traits are very concerned with control. They are preoccupied with trivial details, rules, and order, and because they are perfectionists, they often have difficulty making decisions or getting things done. Such people are usually seen as serious, conventional, stingy, and unbending. If they are obsessive as well, they may be plagued by recurrent and persistent thoughts that they are unable to ignore.

Loss of self-control is the biggest psychological threat to patients with obsessive–compulsive characteristics. Such patients become highly frustrated and anxious if there is any deviation from routine, or changes in their level of control. They react by becoming rigid and indecisive, while seeking more and more information about the illness. These patients usually require little supervision and respond best when given careful, methodical instructions and information, and when allowed to participate in their own medical care.

6.1.3. Histrionic

The characteristics of the histrionic person include an exaggerated expression of emotions, an overreaction to minor events, and a need to constantly draw attention to oneself. Such people are dependent and act helpless. Others consider them to be self-indulgent, demanding, and inconsiderate. Like the borderline, the histrionic person can be prone to manipulative suicidal threats or attempts.

Those diagnosed as histrionic experience physical illness as a threat to masculinity or femininity. Such patients are very dramatic and intense in their personal interactions and may rush headlong into situations, such as medical procedures, without sufficient understanding of the treatment or its consequences. Psychological interventions should include reassurance, support for the patient's attractiveness or physical prowess, and an opportunity to express feelings.

6.1.4. Narcissistic

Narcissistic patients characteristically present themselves as vain, arrogant, and patronizing. They have an exaggerated sense of self-importance and require constant attention and admiration. Yet they experience great shame or feelings of rage when they are unappreciated. There is the feeling of entitlement (i.e., that they are deserving of special favors) without having to respond in kind. They wish to be the center of the universe and would have little empathy for others who are seriously ill.

Their own illness is experienced as a threat to a self-image that is based on autonomy and perfection. In striving for this perfection, narcissistic patients often subject themselves to unnecessary risks by pressing physicians to perform procedures that may not be medically necessary. Those whose illness creates physical impairments or disfigurement would have particular difficulty. Interventions need to support the patient's self-esteem and help rebuild a sense of identity.

6.1.5. Schizoid

Schizoid persons are not interpersonally involved and remain aloof from others. There are usually only one or two people with whom they are even remotely close. Such persons are characterized by an apparent absence of feelings of warmth for others and praise and criticism have little affect on their behavior.

Illness is seen as an intrusion and a threat to the sense of stability they try desperately to maintain. These patients frequently make use of denial and employ withdrawal to keep a comfortable distance from others. Interventions need to respect the desire of these patients for privacy and emotional distance, at the same time helping them comply with the demands of their medical and psychological care, which may be neglected.

6.1.6. Paranoid

Paranoid individuals are suspicious and mistrustful of others. They are hypervigilant, noticing everything around them, and taking special precautions to avoid what they see as possible harm. Since they expect to be tricked, they are guarded and secretive and do not readily accept blame for their own behavior, even when warranted. They also are hypersensitive, exaggerate difficulties, and are easily slighted.

Since paranoid patients are fearful of attack, illness may be experienced as such a feared attack. Physicians' questions may be scrutinized for possible hidden meanings and their motives constantly questioned. The therapist needs to keep some interpersonal distance, recognizing such patients' viewpoint, but being as supporting as possible of procedures necessary for their care that may be looked upon with suspicion.

6.1.7. Hypochondriacal

In 30 to 50% of the visits to primary care physicians, no serious medical disease is found, and 25 to 40% of all patients who are not hospitalized have no diagnosed serious illness. It is expected that about 5% of all medical outpatients have what is commonly referred to as hypochondriasis, i.e., converting emotional distress into physical complaints (Barsky & Klerman, 1985).

Hypochondriacal patients are essentially overconcerned with their own health and bodies. In some cases, patients become obsessively self-conscious following the diagnosis of disease in themselves or in someone they know. Pain, gastrointestinal, cardiac, and respiratory complaints are frequent. This pattern may be temporary or form part of their charac-terological makeup. On the far end of the continuum are those who have a distinct psychiatric disorder in which there is an unrealistic preoccupation with the idea that they have a serious disease (DSM-III). Many of their complaints are vague, ambiguous, or similar to normal bodily sensations ignored by others. Such patients subject themselves to repeated laboratory and surgical procedures, searching for the cause of their illness despite repeated negative findings. It is thought that in some cases these patients benefit psychologically from the attention they receive for their complaints, suggesting an underlying psychiatric problem or a borderline or histrionic personality disorder. In some cases, however, people may be labeled hypo-chondriacs because the physician is simply unable to locate the source of their continued distress. Yet, later, a physical cause for their complaints may be found.

6.2. EMOTIONAL STATES AND ILLNESS

A controversy exists regarding the interaction of emotional states and physical illness (Angell, 1985; Williams, Benson, & Follick, 1985). At pres-ent, the extent to which, and the means by which, psychological and biolog-ical factors interact in the cause, progression, and eventual outcome of illness are not well understood (Livnat & Felten, 1985).

6.2.1. Depression

In a prospective study of male patients on renal dialysis, Ziarnik, Free-man, Sherrard, and Calsyn (1977) found that those who died within one year of initiating dialysis were characterized by feelings of high levels of depression, anxiety, helplessness, and preoccupation with somatic diffi-culties. Those who lived longer were dependent but had milder levels of depression and a sense of hope about the future. But the question remains: Do emotional reactions cause or affect the course of disease, or are they simply a reaction to the illness?

The role of depression in the course of cancer is a case in point. Al-though some recent studies indicate that depression does not correlate with the development of cancer (Streltzer, 1983), the prospective study of over

2000 men at the Western Electric Company in 1957 suggests otherwise (Persky, Kempthorne-Rawson, & Shekelle, 1987). Initially, the men were given the Minnesota Multiphasic Personality Inventory (MMPI). In the 20-year follow-up, 10.5% of the men developed cancer; of that group, 24% had higher scores on the MMPI Depression (D) scale than on the other MMPI scales, as compared with only 18% of the men who did not develop cancer. Also, those scoring higher on the D scale were twice as likely as the average to die of cancer. The actual score differences, however, were quite small. What is of more interest, and probably of more significance, is that the men with the high D scores were more likely to have a family history of cancer. Possibly these men were simply depressed at the time of testing because someone in their family had cancer. The researchers, however, suggest that there may be a genetic factor common to cancer and depression, or that depressed people are more likely to die of cancer because depression suppresses the immune system.

A recent study suggests that the interaction of emotions and illness is more complicated than just which comes first, and reflects possibly a third underlying factor. Lewis *et al.* (1987) discovered a high incidence of mood disorders in women suffering from endometriosis. This condition, which affects about a quarter of the women in their 20s and 30s, is a growth within the pelvic region of tissue normally found only in the lining of the uterus. In their study of 16 women with endometriosis, 12 were found through psychiatric evaluation (interview and testing) to have a history of manic-depressive behavior, meeting the DSM-III criteria for a mood disorder. The rate was higher than expected in the general population. Although cause and effect are not clear here, there is a common link, since both conditions involve abnormal levels of the same hormones.

6.2.2. Anxiety

Rosenman's (1985) discussion of the effects of anxiety on the cardiovascular system illustrates just how intricate the interaction of mind and body is. Although there seems to be a relationship between anxiety and disorders such as arrhythmias, sudden cardiac death, hypertension, and coronary heart disease, it is difficult, at present, to separate cause and effect. Mitral valve prolapse (MVP) is a case in point. Basically, this is a malfunction of the heart valve that occurs frequently in patients with anxiety syndromes. However, patients who suffer from panic attacks that include anxiety, tachycardia, and chest pains are often treated as "neurotic," and the underlying physical disorder (e.g., MVP) is overlooked. On the other hand, panic attacks can result without any evidence of MVP. There is some speculation that MVP and panic attacks, although occasionally occurring together, are different manifestations of a common disorder involving neurotransmitters and hormones.

6.2.3. Anger and Hostility

Anger and hostility appear to have psychological consequences that are related to physical disorders, such as coronary heart disease (CHD), hypertension, and headaches (Chesney & Rosenman, 1985).

Related to this is the body of research that suggests a relationship between coronary heart disease and what has come to be called the Type A personality (e.g., Dembroski & McDougall, 1983; Rosenman, 1985; Rosenman, Brand, Schaltz, & Friedman, 1976). In contrast to the Type B person, who is more relaxed and more accepting of life and others, the Type A person is easily moved to anger, with frequent displays of irritation and hostility. Type A behavior is known as the "hurry sickness" and is characterized by ambitiousness, aggressiveness, competitiveness, and impatience. This pressured behavior has been considered an independent risk factor in coronary disease, of the same magnitude as smoking, a high serum cholesterol level, and hypertension (Review Panel, 1981).

Although most studies have included only male subjects, females, both employed and housewives, exhibit Type A traits. Type A housewives, for example, report poorer marital adjustment and disharmony that do Type Bs. They also report more stress, tension, and physical health problems, fear of failure, and lower self-esteem (Houston & Kelly, 1987).

The research on Type A personalities is controversial, however, since not all studies have found associations between Type A behavior and coronary heart disease. Also, attempts to relate Type A behavior to other diseases has had mixed results (e.g., polio—Bruno & Frick, 1987; peptic ulcer—Langeluddecke, Goulston, & Tennant, 1987). The discrepancies may arise from the different questionnaires and interview techniques used to assess the presence of the Type A pattern. Or, the relationship, if it exists, may be more complicated than previously thought, and thus not always easy to measure (Case, Heller, Case, Moss, et al., 1985; Dimsdale, 1988; Fischman, 1987; Ragland & Brand, 1988; Shekelle et al., 1985).

Researchers who have tried to understand the components of personality that affect illness have found hostility (as measured by the Ho scale of the MMPI) to be more predictive of heart attack and survival than the global Type A assessments (Barefoot, Dahlstrom, & Williams, 1983; Williams et al., 1980). Studies using other scales reveal that hostility itself takes many forms, which interact differently with coronary artery disease. Persons who quite readily express anger and annoyance have been found to be at risk for CHD (Siegman, Dembroski, & Ringel, 1987), as do those who are cynical and not trusting of others. According to Wright's recent analyses (1988), there are at least five separate routes to CHD, with the strongest factors being (a) denial and consciously controlled anger directed inward—i.e., the person feels it is inappropriate to express anger or just cannot do it; and (b) anger directed outward, in combination with time urgency and chronic activation. Additional risk factors include the traditional global Type A behavior pattern; certain non-Type A behaviors, such as smoking, poor diet, and poor exercise habits; and a family history of CHD.

Studies reveal that the traits of anger, hostility, cynicism, and suspiciousness affect a person's tendency to succumb to other disorders, as well as heart attacks (Barefoot *et al.*, 1983; Berkman & Syme, 1979; Ruberman, Weinblatt, Goldber, & Chaudhary, 1984). Persons with these characteristics are understandably socially isolated and under stress. Current research is focusing on the interaction of social support networks and coronary artery disease, but results, although suggestive of a positive relationship between support and CHD for Type A's, are at present inconclusive (Blumenthal *et al.*, 1987; Cohen & Matthews, 1987; Seeman & Syme, 1987). Despite all the research, two basic, but related, questions remain: (1) To what extent do personality traits "cause" disease, and to what extent are they a result of patients' attempts to adapt to a chronic illness (Moran, 1985)? (2) Are there certain personality types associated with specific diseases, or is there a general "disease-prone personality"?

6.3. The Disease-Prone Personality: Does It Exist?

For centuries both physicians and laymen have hypothesized that certain personalities have a predisposition toward specific diseases. Tuberculosis, for example, was romantically associated with writers, poets, and artists, whose supposed predisposing characteristics were that they were passionate and repressed (Sontag, 1979). The picture began to change in the late 19th century, when it was demonstrated that TB was contagious and caused by a bacillus. But even this scientific finding did not totally explain why some individuals who had been exposed to the illness did not develop the disease.

In the 1940s and 1950s, the subject of the relationship between tuberculosis and personality was revived (Hartz, 1944, 1950; Holmes *et al.*, 1957). Although researchers found evidence of stress and conflicts over dependency in tubercular patients, there was no actual evidence for a "tuberculosis-prone personality."

Over the years, other illnesses, such as cancer, diabetes, rheumatoid arthritis, and dermatological disorders, have also been attributed to specific psychological traits and life events (Cassileth *et al.*, 1984; Pow, 1987; Scurry & Levin, 1978–1979; Streltzer, 1983). The "diabetic personality" was described as depressed and apathetic, suffering from stress. Willis, a 17th-century physician, boldly attributed diabetes to "an ill manner of living…sadness, long grief" (cited in Major, 1965). The "arthritic personality" was described as depressed, repressed, anxious, and stressful. Ulcers were thought to be related to oral conflicts, migraine headaches to repressed hostility, and asthma to separation anxiety (e.g., Alexander, 1950). What is striking about these "predisposing" personality syndromes is how similar they are. One difficulty is that each body of literature describes personality traits as though they applied only to the illnesses under study, without making reference to patients with other diseases who show similar traits.

Cassileth *et al.* (1984) set out to investigate the question of personality and medical illness, focusing on patients with arthritis, diabetes, cancer, renal disease, and dermatological disorders. The researchers found that patients with various diseases did not differ in their psychological reactions. And in fact, their psychological profile was similar to that of the public in general, and was much healthier than that of a group of patients under treatment for psychiatric depression. Overall, the patients' mental health was poorer during the first three months after diagnosis, as compared with later on, reflecting difficulties in initially adjusting to the shock of diagnosis, the initial physical symptoms, and the treatment regimens. Severity of illness was associated with poorer mental health, with those having the more disabling conditions or in the advanced stages of disease showing more depression and other psychological problems.

Although specific personality characteristics may not lead to specific illnesses, Friedman and Booth-Kewley (1987) concluded from their analyses of current research that there may be a "generic disease-prone personality" that is depressed, angry, hostile, and anxious. These researchers conducted a meta-analysis of 229 studies, covering 1945 to 1984. Combining studies investigating similar factors, they arrived at overall correlations ranging from about .10 to .25 between personality problems (i.e., depression, anxiety, hostility) and disease (i.e., chronic heart disease, asthma, ulcer, arthritis, and headache). The strongest relationship was between the personality variables and heart disease. Correlation coefficients of this magnitude, however, do not explain a large proportion of the variance, and they suggest that these emotional factors are only a small part of the larger picture. But, as the researchers point out, when one is dealing with large populations, even a small relationship may be indicative of something affecting thousands of individuals. However, a meta-analysis is only as good as the research upon which it is based, and as the researchers themselves mention, their evidence for a disease-prone personality is weak in light of the small correlations, and the fact that most of the studies included in the analysis were retrospective and had relatively small sample sizes.

6.4. Stress and the Immune System

But what about the emotions as causative factors in illness? The psychological syndrome of anger and hostility and that of depression, anxiety, and repression have similar physiological consequences (i.e., elevated levels of corticosteroids and catecholamines), which have been associated with immunosuppression and metabolic abnormalities (e.g., Jemmot & Locke, 1984; Krantz, Baum, & Singer, 1983). Although the exact mechanisms are not understood, extensive reviews of the literature lead to the conclusion that stress results in decreased immune system functioning, which in turn can lead to disease (Ader, 1981; Baker, 1987; Jemmot & Locke, 1984; S. Levy, 1985; Solomon, 1985). The effect of stress may be transient and limited, having the most serious consequences for those with preexisting deficits in immune functioning—for example, the elderly, patients with immunosuppressive diseases such as AIDS, or those who have been exposed to an infectious agent or carcinogen (Kiecolt-Glaser & Glaser, 1986).

Stress has been shown to inhibit the ability of lymphocytes and macrophages to destroy tumors in both animals (Pavlidis & Chirigos, 1980) and humans (Bartrop, Lazarus, Luckhurst, Kiloh, & Penny, 1977). However, studies with animals have revealed an ability to adapt gradually to the effects of stress, making them less vulnerable to its tumor-enhancing effects (Sklar, Bruto, & Anisman, 1981). And in certain situations, stress itself has been shown to inhibit tumor growth (Sklar & Anisman, 1981).

6.4.1. Life Events

It is commonly assumed nowadays that life events, particularly those that are stressful, may predispose one to serious illness. In one study, for example, men who developed lung cancer, as compared with those who had benign lung lesions, were more likely to have had a recent significant loss and to lack plans for the future (Horne & Picard, 1979). Paradoxically, they also had more job stability, a situation that should counteract, to some extent, stresses in life. In another study, stressful, uncontrollable life events in the past year were related to the advent of chest pain in patients who did not have coronary heart disease (Roll & Theorell, 1987). These patients also received high scores on measures of Type A personality. Their chest pains were thought to be related to the interaction of psychological factors and the body (e.g., muscle tension, respiration).

Most studies in this area, however, have methodological problems, and data available show little relationship between the life events and stress (Scurry & Levin, 1978–1979). In evaluating stress, one needs to consider what aspects of life events are stressful, the amount of change required, the desirability of the event, the ability to understand what is happening, and the extent to which the event was expected or controllable (Cronkite & Moos, 1984).

6.4.2. Reactions to Stress

Some studies have suggested that it is not stress *per se* that triggers the disease course but the way in which the individual reacts to, or copes with, the stressor. In a study of those with abnormal cervical cells (Goodkin,

Antoni, & Blaney, 1986), development of cancer was associated with two factors: (a) premorbid pessimism, defined as the tendency to interpret life as a series of troubles and misfortunes, along with an attitude of helplessness and hopelessness; and (b) an inhibited copying style, defined as fearful, distrustful, and shy, keeping problems "inside," and exhibiting low self-esteem. Analysis of the data suggests that both factors must be present to affect the course of the disease. This is an important point, since research often looks at isolated aspects of the person's psychosocial world without understanding their interactions or putting them into perspective in terms of their overall importance. Caution should be used, however, when generalizing from the Goodkin *et al.* study because the results were based on small samples. Also, patients in the more advanced stages of the disease were assessed while in the hospital; those not so ill were in an outpatient clinic. The different environments alone would be expected to affect a person's responses to questions about stress and thus confound the results of the study.

If stress is considered a cause of disease, then patients can experience a sense of hope if they feel they can control their destiny, either by preventing illness or by helping themselves to get better. However, if sickness does occur, or if the disease spreads despite great efforts toward positive thinking and living, then patients must deal with the guilt that they themselves are responsible for their own sickness. This feeling of responsibility (based on an assumption yet to be proven) is an added burden that the sick person must bear (Angell, 1985). There are, however, some patients who prefer to feel the responsibility despite the guilt, since the sense of control over their own fate is more acceptable than dealing with the unknown, or blaming others or God.

6.5. CONCLUSIONS

Some people still hold to the idea that those having certain personality types are more likely to get one illness over another. This, however, has not been borne out by current research, with the possible exception of certain traits associated with the Type A personality and heart disease. What appears to be the case is that patients are likely to react emotionally to the stresses of serious illness *per se*, rather than reacting in certain ways to one disease as compared with another. Research suggests that patients with different diseases share traits in common (e.g., depression, anxiety, feelings of hopelessness and helplessness), and that these emotions are a reaction to the illness rather than a precipitant. Certain patients cope with physical illness in the way that they typically cope with other stressful life experiences. Along with this is the growing evidence that, in some instances, biochemical and hormonal changes play a role, affecting both the course of the illness and a person's emotional reactions.

Although an individual's psychological characteristics do not appear to make the person more susceptible to one disease over another, emotional makeup can be a contributing factor, especially if it results in stress or unhealthful behavior. Anxiety, for example, can lead people to overeat, exacerbating hypertension, diabetes, and other conditions. Depression can lead to use of drugs, which can affect the central nervous system, for example, or to the use of alcohol, which in excess can affect the central nervous system and the liver, and even in moderation has been implicated in breast cancer (Graham, 1987; Schatzkin *et al.*, 1987; Willett *et al.*, 1987). And various social psychological factors lead a person to smoke cigarettes, which in turn cause cancer, heart disease, and respiratory conditions. Essentially, psychological factors are but one of a number of interacting variables (biological, psychological, and sociological) that determine how a disease develops in each individual (Stoudemire, 1985).

7

Sex and Sexuality

7.1. CARDIOVASCULAR DISEASE

The physical requirements for sexual intercourse have been compared to those for "a brisk walk around a city block" (Wise, 1983). Most patients with uncomplicated myocardial infarction (MI, heart attack) have the capacity for twice that expenditure of energy. Despite this, a significant number of men and women have sexual difficulties following a heart attack. As many as 60% of the men in one study reported erectile difficulties, and a third premature ejaculation (Mehta & Krop, 1979). Although medication or the complications of a heart attack could inhibit sexual functioning, in most cases it appears to be related to depression and anxiety. A certain amount of depression or lack of desire is to be expected during the recovery period following a heart attack or surgery. But if the lack of interest continues for more than a few months, other medical or psychological factors may be involved. For one, the medication may need to be adjusted. In some cases, patients who still experience the pain of angina may be disappointed with their recovery, and this may lead to the continuing depression.

Following a heart attack, a patient is usually instructed to refrain from sexual intercourse for a month or two. Then, gradual resumption of sexual contact, such as touching and stroking, is suggested to help overcome any sexual inhibitions that may have resulted, as well as to test out the physiological effects. Following a bypass operation, for example, pain from the incision may be confused with an early sign of heart attack. Patients may need to change positions during intercourse to minimize weight-bearing on the operative site. Patients do need to be alert, however, to serious symptoms, such as pressure, pain, or discomfort in the jaw, neck, arm, chest, or stomach; marked shortness of breath; and excessively rapid or irregular heartbeat (Resuming Sex after Heart Surgery, 1987). These symptoms should be brought to the immediate attention of the physician.

Those who have suffered a stroke (cerebral accident) may find that they engage in sexual intercourse less frequently. This may be related to actual physical limitations resulting from the stroke, but frequently the problem is compounded by the psychological effect of these limitations on the person's self-image (Sjogren & Fugl-Meyer, 1982).

7.2. Kidney Disease

The incidence of sexual problems is higher in patients with kidney disease (ESRD; end stage renal disease) than in the "general" population (N.B. Levy, 1981, 1984; Levy & Wyntraub, 1975; Mine, Golden, & Fibus, 1978). After the start of dialysis, as compared with the preceding uremic period, there is usually a reduction in the frequency of intercourse and of orgasm, and an increase in impotence. For example, 59% of the men studied by Levy (1984) reported difficulty, either totally or partially, having an erection. Renal transplantation seems to improve sexual functioning, but not to the level of functioning prior to the illness (Procci, Hoffman, & Chatterjee, 1978).

Woodburne (1973) found that 70% of the patients he studied did have intercourse at some time following the onset of kidney failure. However, the majority reported a decrease in the frequency of their sexual activity. Of interest was that the patients tended to report a decrease more often than their spouses did. Why this difference in perception? Possibly patients' depression or unmet needs clouded their memory, or spouses were giving socially acceptable answers or denying to themselves the extent of sexual deprivation.

The underlying reasons for sexual problems in kidney disease seem to be primarily organic, and related to the hormonal system. Antihypertensive medications are a contributing factor as well. Compounding the problem is that patients on dialysis tend to be chronically anemic and, because of the diminished strength and energy, become less interested in sexual intercourse. The self-image also is involved, since kidney failure can lead to the cessation of menstruation and urination, which may be experienced as a loss of sexuality. And reproductive capacity may be affected, making it difficult for unmarried individuals to find a stable mate (Binik, 1983).

One way to distinguish between the organic and the psychological basis of sexual problems in men is to measure nocturnal penile tumescence (NPT). It has been observed that men experience erections during phase one REM sleep. By measuring changes in penile circumference during the night, the examiner can ascertain whether the individual has the ability to have erections. Studies have reported that the patients with advanced uremic conditions and those on hemodialysis have significantly shorter mean NPT times, as compared with others of the same age and those with chronic physical conditions who are not uremic (Levy, 1984). These findings support the theory that organic factors play a primary role in the sexual problems of patients with kidney disease.

7.3. DIABETES

Diabetes is probably the most common organic cause of male sexual dysfunction and is the side effect of greatest concern to diabetic men (Jensen, 1981; Podolsky, 1982). From 40 to 50% of adult males with diabetes experience some type of sexual dysfunction, the most prevalent being erectile difficulties (Cox, Gonder-Frederick, Pohl, & Pennebaker, 1986). The problem has a gradual onset and appears to be related to peripheral and autonomic neurological problems, rather than to diabetic severity, type of diabetes, or medication.

For many men, diabetic impotence is the result of an interaction between psychological and organic factors. In a study of 60 reportedly impotent diabetic men (Abel, Becker, Cunningham-Rathner, Mittelman, & Primack, 1982), 28% were able to have erections during sleep, suggesting a psychological basis for their impotence. As with other impotent males, this study suggests that complete psychological and organic evaluations need to be conducted before a diagnosis is made. In some cases, surgical prosthetic implants might be indicated, but they are expensive and involve a certain amount of psychological and physical risk. Since 60% of those diagnosed as having organic impotence do in fact improve their sexual functioning with traditional sex therapy (Abel *et al.*, 1982), sex therapy should be attempted first and should be a part of treatment even when the cause is considered organically based.

Sexual dysfunction does not appear to be a major problem for diabetic women (Jensen, 1981), although early studies did report orgasmic dysfunction due to neurological problems and degenerative vascular changes (Kolodny, 1971). Diabetic women, however, are susceptible to vaginal infections and dyspareunia (painful intercourse), especially when blood glucose levels are high (Krosnick & Podolsky, 1981). Oral contraceptives and interuterine devices are contraindicated, so other methods need to be used (Campbell & McCulloch, 1979). Fertility may be impaired as well. Those who become pregnant may experience a more rapid progression of the illness—for example, more eye problems (retinopathy). Also, there is a higher probability of perinatal mortality and congenital abnormalities if one or both parents are diabetic. The offspring of diabetic parents, however, are not at great risk for developing diabetes, i.e., 10% if one parent and 20% if both parents are diabetic (Cox *et al.*, 1986).

7.4. ILEOSTOMY AND COLOSTOMY

Negative body image, lowered self-esteem, and fear of injury contribute to the decrease in frequency of intercourse reported for both men and women who have undergone an ileostomy or a colostomy. There is often a concern about odors and spillage, or fear that the bag will slip off during intercourse. Adolescents and unmarried adults may become socially withdrawn because they worry about dating and future sexual performance.

In males, sexual functioning is impaired in about 50% of the colostomy patients and in almost all patients after bladder removal (Kirkpatrick, 1980). Women frequently experience dyspareunia (painful intercourse) if the disease process affects the rectum (Brook, 1979). Decreased fertility has also been noted for women with ostomies; however, the reason is unknown. A cooperative and understanding partner is helpful in assisting with the coping process, and sexual functioning does appear to improve over time (Wise, 1983). But should a relationship begin to deteriorate, the patient or partner may find it more difficult to be accepting of the ostomy and focus on it as the source of stress, overlooking psychodynamic or interpersonal factors that are at the root of the problem.

7.5. CANCER

Since cancer often strikes the sexual organs, its affect on sexual functioning is of great importance. Not only does the tumor have its devastating effects but treatment (e.g., surgery and radiation) can be disfiguring and destructive of function. Treatment for diseases such as urological cancer, for example, can destroy the physical integrity of sexual organs, interfering radically with patients' customary ways of achieving physical pleasure and intimacy, and lessening their sense of personal worth (Schover, von Eschenbach, Smith, & Gonzales, 1984). Sexual therapy is required in such cases for patients to learn new ways of achieving physical pleasure, and options, such as prostheses, may need to be discussed.

Gynecological surgery may involve the removal of the vaginal wall; however, patients have reported resuming a "satisfying" sexual life despite difficulties with orgasm (Morley, Lindenaver, & Youngs, 1973). When patients with breast or gynecological cancer did report sexual difficulties, these tended to persist and did not resolve themselves if left untreated (Andersen & Jochimsen, 1985). Some of the psychological problems developed almost immediately, and others as much as a year or two later. When a patient is given the diagnosis of breast cancer, for example, she must deal with the threat of death, pain, and disfigurement, and the potential loss of sexuality. Although shame and embarrassment may occur as a result of scarring and the change in body image, the vast majority of breast cancer patients apparently make a satisfactory recovery (Andersen & Jochimsen, 1985; Meyerowitz, Sparks, & Spears, 1979).

The results of studies of the sexual difficulties of cancer patients, however, are mixed (Andersen & Jochimsen, 1985, 1987; Thomas, 1987). Differences are dependent upon the site and stage of the illness, the extent of treatment, the definition of sexual dysfunction, and the statistical methodology used in each study.

7.6. Seizure Disorder

There are many possible causes of the abnormality referred to as a seizure disorder: birth defects, head injuries, diseases such as measles or encephalitis, disorders of the circulatory system, and tumors. In many cases, the cause is not known. Although the disorder does not affect a person's sexual functioning organically, it can interfere with sexual relationships. If the seizures are not controlled, fear about the possibility of having a seizure during intercourse can inhibit sexual performance and pleasure.

Not so long ago there were laws in some states forbidding those with epilepsy to marry. Even today, without such laws, the individuals themselves still must deal with questions regarding marriage and having children. One issue is the fear that a severely handicapped person may not be able to care for a child. The concern about having a seizure while taking care of a child is real; for those whose seizures are controlled by medication, however, this should pose little or no problem.

Another issue is the fear that the child will also become epileptic. Although some irregular brain-wave patterns may run in families, epilepsy is not generally considered to be a genetically transmitted disease. Research suggests, however, that children born to epileptic mothers have an increased risk of cleft lip and palate. Most studies have looked at data only from mothers; however, Friis (1979) reported an increased risk if either parent were epileptic.

The risks involved in the interaction of anticonvulsants and seizures on pregnancy are only beginning to be understood. According to the Epilepsy Foundation of America (1985), at least 90% of women with epilepsy who take anticonvulsant medication during pregnancy give birth to normal, healthy infants. However, in recent years research suggests that taking seizure-preventing drugs during pregnancy increases the risk of birth defects. The risk appears to be about two to three times the normal rate, and possibly higher for some drugs (Kaplan & Wyler, 1983).

A study of 902 pregnant women in Japan investigated the interaction of seizures and medication during pregnancy (Nakane et al., 1980). The authors reported that fetal malformations were lowest in women who were unmedicated and who had no seizures during pregnancy. The highest incidence were in those who were taking medication, and who also had seizures. The greatest risk was with a drug called Trimethadione. The highest risk phase is, however, during the first trimester, and many women find out they are pregnant only after this period.

Such research presents women with a conflict. If they discontinue the drugs during pregnancy, they run the risk of having a seizure; this risk is real, since some women have more seizures during pregnancy than at other times. Also, having a seizure while pregnant could have deleterious effects on the fetus by depriving it of oxygen because of the mother's impaired breathing, or injuring the fetus should the mother fall.

7.7. ASTHMA

Those with severe or chronic asthma often have a diminution of sexual desire (Thompson & Thompson, 1985). Lack of energy due to physiological and psychological factors can make sex a lesser priority. Also, because of their condition they may be excused from normal activities, which can include being a sexual partner. In some cases, the increased respiratory rate during sexual activity may be mistaken for asthmatic dyspnea (shortness of breath). This can lead to anxiety and can provoke an actual asthma attack. In addition, many asthmatics cannot tolerate exercise and may develop bronchial spasms from sexual activity. Although this can usually be treated with adrenergic medication given prior to sexual activity, many patients do not discuss their sexual difficulties with their physicians, choosing to avoid sex instead.

7.8. INTERPERSONAL FACTORS AFFECTING SEXUALITY

Extreme weight loss, unsightly scars from accidents or operations, and paralysis all affect the self-concept and, as a result, sexuality. Often it is the patients themselves who pull away from the intimacy, feeling that they can no longer be responsive, and wanting no part of a physical relationship.

The impersonal attitude of the medical environment also can negatively affect sexuality.

> Maida found that she shied away from her fiancé for months following her extended treatments. During physical examinations, she felt naked and exposed. Her body had been looked at and handled by so many strangers that she no longer felt like a sexual being. She had kept her sexual feelings in check to such an extent that she now had difficulty presenting herself as beautiful and mysterious. Being close to her fiancé was no longer stimulating. She felt nothing, and at times even found the idea of sex repulsive.

Another complicating problem is that many healthy people act as though sick people are asexual and have no sexual feelings. The patient begins to accept the idea that there is something wrong about "thinking about such things at a time like this." Physicians may reinforce this attitude because they measure success in terms of survival. They are more likely to be concerned with prolonging life and controlling the disease than with the quality of the life *per se*. Yet sometimes physicians hide behind their ultimate mission because they, like much of the population, are embarrassed about sexual matters. As a result, they assume that a person's sex life is satisfactory if the patient does not bring it up. When sexual dysfunction is identified, it may be attributed to disease-related causes, and the psychological problems of the patient or the patient's spouse may be overlooked (Anderson & Wolf, 1986). The following example illustrates how psychodynamic and interpersonal issues can affect a patient's sex life and become intertwined with the illness in complicated ways.

After Max's 40-year-old wife, Bea, had her first heart attack, she withdrew emotionally and physically. She became very depressed and also fearful of any strenuous activity. Although her physician had made no sexual restrictions, she refused to have intercourse with Max. (Actually, their sex life prior to her illness had not been good, and it is likely that Bea used this opportunity to distance herself even more from her husband.)

Now, 10 years after Bea's death, Max is in psychotherapy for his own depression following the diagnosis of lymphoma. He talks hesitantly about his infidelity during the period of his wife's illness and the guilt he still feels. And he cringes as he hears himself, a 70-year-old man, saying, "I just had those urges. Bea wouldn't sleep with me. I was a young man." But the guilt eats away at him as he thinks of his wife and how he misses her, of how he would like her to be with him, to take care of him, to comfort him.

Long-standing interpersonal psychodynamic issues may need to be dealt with in therapy. Infidelity, for example, can cause internal conflict if the caretaker has found a sex life outside the marriage. There may be suppressed anger toward the ill spouse for deserting the healthy partner, not only sexually but through illness and later death. There may be guilt toward the new sexual partner, who presses for a closer relationship, as well as guilt toward the ill spouse as a result of the deceit. The unfaithful spouse may interpret any later difficulties as a punishment for the waywardness.

7.9. Psychological Intervention

Psychotherapy can play a major role in improving the sexual life of the medically ill, through minimizing misunderstandings and problems that may emerge. Often, for example, patients and their families are under the mistaken impression that sexual activity may cause increased risks for the ill person and, thus, they refrain from any form of intimacy (Schover *et al.*, 1984). As medically indicated, the therapist can provide counseling and suggestions for the resumption of sexual activity, but this should be appropriate to the patient's attitudes and patterns of sexual expression prior to the illness. Often a gradual return to sexual activity is recommended following a serious illness. During this period, the participants can rediscover sensu-

ality by focusing on touching, stroking, body massage, and other alternatives to traditional sexual intercourse (Anderson & Wolf, 1986). Even simple
physical contact, such as bathing, manicuring nails, or hand-holding, can
be experienced as sensual and allow the sick person to feel attractive and
cared for. Therapists counseling on sexual techniques need to keep in contact with the patient's physician, so the methods suggested do not compromise the patient physically.

8

Suicide

Suicidal thoughts are a function of feelings of hopelessness and helplessness (Shneidman, 1978). Underlying these thoughts are a host of fears, often related to issues of loss. The patient may fear the possibility of loss of function or sight, or even life itself. There is the fear of losing love and affection, or one's attractiveness, as a result of an illness. And there is the fear of having contracted a disease, such as AIDS, with the possibility of pain and suffering or social disgrace. Suicide can also be triggered by an underlying emotional disturbance, such as a clinical depression or a personality disorder. Or it may be related to a central nervous system disorder, stemming from the physical effects of the disease itself, or the treatment.

When working with the physically ill, one needs to differentiate between irrationally motivated noncompliance or denial of illness (such as managing one's medical condition inconsistently and/or destructively) and behavior or thoughts that are unrelated to a mental disorder (such as concern that treatment and the quality of life may be worse than death itself).

8.1. THE FUNCTION OF SUICIDAL IDEATION

Suicidal thoughts are not uncommon in those with severe disabilities or deteriorating illnesses (Clark, Cavanaugh, & Gibbons, 1983). A patient may begin to "feel like a burden" or that others would be "better off without me." Many do not speak openly about such thoughts because of the social stigma attached to suicide. Some who do talk about wishing to die, or who contemplate suicide, may do so out of despair or to gain needed attention or pity.

In the more emotionally intact patients, who constitute the vast majority, the contemplation of suicide can be seen as an attempt to regain control. With everything out of their power and the future unknown, the idea that they might be able to end it is one of the last remaining areas in which they feel they can still exercise some control. This does not mean that they will actually try to kill themselves, only that they need to feel that there is a way out, an option that they could exercise if need be—an option that few, even those who suffer greatly, choose to take.

It is important to provide an atmosphere where the individual is free to discuss the suicidal feelings. Typically, many believe that the therapist needs to be clearly aligned as an advocate for remaining alive and coping with disease. However, this should not take the form of judging or moralizing, or suggesting that the patient is "crazy" if he or she openly discusses the desire to die. Threats of hospitalization may come from the professional's own panic and fear that things are getting out of control. And premature threats of psychiatric hospitalization can be experienced as punishment for "being bad," rather than as a protective measure for the patient's benefit. Patients may pull away and sink further into depression at the idea that their last avenue of escape is being taken away.

Discussing the issue seriously and comfortably and acknowledging the patient's psychic and physical pain can be consoling. Also, explaining that thoughts of death are not uncommon for seriously ill or disabled persons can be reassuring.

8.2. SUICIDE THREATS

Suicide threats may be used to manipulate others, to punish, or to express anger and hostility (Boehnert & Popkin, 1986). Some patients with underlying personality disorders thrive on the interpersonal conflict they create, and use the illness and threats of suicide for their own purposes. When working with such patients, therapists need to be consistent in their approach, firm in setting limits, and direct when discussing self-harm attempts. They also need to maintain a sufficient distance from dramatic "rescue" maneuvers and the chaos with which these patients surround themselves.

Although in some cases hospitalization may be indicated, with more intact patients it is possible to work with their ego strengths and basic desire to survive: to listen, to be understanding, and to help the person through the difficult and (one hopes) transient period. Exploring the issue and what it would mean to the patient and to others helps to defuse the immediacy of the thought. It also lets the patients know that their despair and fears are being taken seriously.

8.3. SUICIDE ATTEMPTS

For the population at large the probability of actually committing suicide is low, i.e., about 12 persons in 100,000 per year (U.S. Bureau of the

Census, 1985), and the vast majority of these cases are severely emotionally disturbed. However, having a serious medical illness may add additional stress, causing certain individuals to be at more risk than others (Clark et al., 1983).

A study by Farberow, Ganzler, Cutter, and Reynolds (1971) conducted with hospitalized VA patients found suicides in neuropsychiatric hospitals to be six times higher than in the general population, while in the general medical and surgical hospitals the risk was much lower, by almost half. After age 50, however, the medical diagnoses begin to outnumber the neuropsychiatric diagnoses in number of suicide cases. Slightly more than half of the suicidal medical patients actually committed suicide while they were in the hospital, usually by jumping out a window or hanging themselves. Outside the hospital, guns were the most common means. It should be kept in mind, however, that the vast majority of patients in this study were males, and males generally are reported to use more violent (and effective) means when attempting suicide. Also, the study did not control for possible underlying psychiatric illness in the medical population.

When assessing the medical seriousness of a suicide attempt, one needs to consider the *risk*, which refers to the actual dangerousness of the attempt, and the *rescue fantasy*, which refers to the possible desire of the person to be saved (Weisman & Worden, 1972). In addition, clinicians should be alert for signs of alcoholism and drug abuse, which are often contributing factors (Fischer, Knop, & Graem, 1985; Flavin, Franklin, & Frances, 1986; Whitfield, 1984).

Other risk factors may include (a) preexisting emotional disturbance, (b) family and financial problems, (c) reduced tolerance for pain, (d) threats of self-destruction, (e) severe depression, coupled with clear thinking, and (f) attempts to control treatment (Farberow, Shneidman, & Leonard, 1963).

8.4. MEDICAL ILLNESSES: RISK FACTORS

Reliable statistics on suicide are difficult to come by. It is estimated that suicides may be underreported by as much as 22% (Schoenfeld et al., 1984). Available data are confounded by the social stigma attached to the act, accidental deaths, and so-called "passive" suicides. For example, if the effects of chemotherapy are severe, some patients may refuse to undergo continued treatments, fully aware that death may be a consequence of their decision (Burish & Lyles, 1983; Seigel & Longo, 1981; Whitehead, 1975). Is this suicide? In cases of advancing disease, "giving up" or not cooperating may reflect the disease process itself, rather than being a cause of death.

8.4.1. Cancer

Cancer is often seen as the prototype of the fatal illness, representing the extremes in pain and prolonged suffering. Yet the vast majority of those so afflicted do not wish for death or choose to take their own lives. In fact, research is mixed about the extent to which suicide is prevalent among cancer patients. Some studies suggest that the rate of suicide may be no greater, or even less, than in the general population (Siegel & Tuckel, 1984–1985), while others have found a high incidence.

Marshall, Burnett, and Brasure (1983) reported that cancer patients are 50 to 100% more likely to commit suicide than nonpatients. And in an earlier study, Farberow *et al.* (1971) found that patients with neoplastic disease constituted 23% of the 171 medical patients who had committed suicide over an eight-year period. Since these patients represented only 11% of the hospital patients, they were overrepresented in the suicide group, suggesting a greater risk for suicide in cancer patients than in those with some other diseases.

Plumb and Holland (1981) found that cancer patients had better psychological adjustment prior to their illness than a comparison group made up of nonphysically ill persons who had attempted suicide. At the time of illness, a third of the cancer patients in their study manifested overt depression. Roughly a seventh were experiencing suicidal ideation, which was rated as mild to moderate in severity. Typically, these thoughts were linked to moderate rather than severe depression. Cancer patients who expressed suicidal thoughts took comfort in the idea that if things got worse, "I could always kill myself." Thus, having an escape route from pain and deterioration may have acted to relieve depression. Others chose not to kill themselves because of not wanting to hurt loved ones who would survive.

A history of prior depressive episodes and a tendency to brood in the past were characteristics that distinguished the cancer patients who had severe depression from those who did not. This suggests that the stress of a current illness may exacerbate a preexisting affective disorder or characterological depressive trait.

Research is mixed on identifying when in the course of the disease the patient is most vulnerable. Excess risk of suicide appears to occur within the first five years after diagnosis (Louhivuori & Hakama, 1979) and in the later stages of the disease (Farberow, 1981; Holland, 1977). Suicidal thoughts may be prevalent when the illness is first diagnosed or following recurrence (Silberfarb, Mauer, & Crouthamel, 1980). Families and physicians are often afraid that patients will commit suicide if told they have cancer. Although accurate data are not available, a survey of 219 physicians revealed only two cases where the patient committed suicide shortly after having been given the diagnosis of cancer (Oken, 1961). And in another study, only 10 of the 44 terminally ill hospitalized patients interviewed wished for death, and only 3 of these admitted having considered suicide (Brown, Henteleff, Barakat, & Rowe, 1986).

Suicide is more likely to occur in those with poorer psychological resources and less ability to adjust to illness (Farberow et al., 1963). Other patient characteristics associated with higher risk for cancer patients are the following:

1. *Marital status*—divorced and never married patients (particularly women) having a higher risk (Louhivuori & Hakama, 1979; Marshall et al., 1983).
2. *Extent of disease*—those whose disease has spread being at twice the risk as those whose disease is localized (Louhivuori & Hakama, 1979).
3. *Treatment*—those receiving chemotherapy or palliation being at increased risk (Louhivuori & Hakama, 1979).
4. *Age*—young patients and those over age 60 being at greater risk (Farberow, 1981).
5. *Site*—increased risk being associated with gastrointestinal cancers (Farberow, 1981) and cancer of the brain, face, pancreas, lung, larynx, and tongue (Farberow et al., 1971).

8.4.2. Epilepsy

A review of the literature reveals that the suicide rate for those with epilepsy is from four to seven times that expected of the population at large (Brent, 1986; Hawton, Fagg, & Marsack, 1980; MacKay, 1979; Matthews & Barabas, 1981).

Factors that may interact to cause a person with a seizure disorder to attempt suicide are (a) the chronicity of the illness, (b) the neuropsychiatric effects of the epilepsy, (c) family stressors, (d) social stigma and its ramifications, (e) iatrogenic effects of anticonvulsant medication, and (f) the constant availability of drugs (Batzel & Dodrill, 1986). Studies of epileptic patients have reported an association between suicidal behavior and the use of phenobarbital (Hawton et al., 1980; MacKay, 1979; Prudhomme, 1941). This drug can cause depression and have a negative effect on feelings of self-esteem. The availability of drugs prescribed for seizures constitutes a particular hazard, since the incidence of self-poisoning in epilepsy is seven times that in the general population (MacKay, 1979). In addition, suicide attempters have reported experiencing three times as much stress as psychiatric patients who were not suicidal (Luscomb, Clum, & Patsiokas, 1980). Brain lesions and frequent and severe seizures are also thought to be risk factors (Green & Mercille, 1984).

Sex differences also emerge. As is the case in the general population, three times as many women as men with epilepsy attempt suicide, with the men using more violent means and being more successful (Batzel & Dodrill, 1986).

8.4.3. Acquired Immune Deficiency Syndrome (AIDS)

The stressors for this disease include (a) the unknown and dreaded course of the disease, (b) the absence of cure, (c) social isolation, and (d) guilt and fear regarding sexual transmission (Flavin *et al.*, 1986). Despite the pervasiveness of the disease, the suicide rate does not appear to be high. This may be due, in part, to the networks for psychological counseling and support services that have evolved. However, given that AIDS is a communicable disease, patients' behavior is of great concern.

Attempting to contract a communicable disease is a subtle form of suicidal behavior that may escape recognition. Anecdotal accounts of such behavior in the past have been associated with tuberculosis, polio, and syphilis (Flavin *et al.*, 1986). Now there are clinical accounts of persons who have actively tried to contract AIDS (Frances, Wikstrom, & Alcena, 1985; Flavin *et al.*, 1986). The extent of this behavior is currently unknown; however, with the growing number of AIDS cases, therapists need to be alert to the possibility of such behavior, particularly with emotionally disturbed individuals.

Clinical case studies suggest that depression, sexual conflicts, and narcissistic and histrionic personality disorders may be underlying factors. Catching the disease may be perceived as more acceptable than actively committing suicide. The patients may have tried suicide unsuccessfully, may be afraid of using violent or unsuccessful means, or may not want to upset their family because of the social stigma attached to the act. One patient, described by Flavin *et al.* (1986), saw the disease as a convenient and dramatic way to die, while being cared for in the process. Also, angry, hostile patients have expressed the wish to transmit the disease to others. In either case, such patients have been known to continue to engage in anonymous, unprotected sex, until the underlying motivations have been confronted and worked through in therapy.

8.4.4. Diabetes

"Cheating, excessive denial, pathological family dynamics and fear of complications affect the patient's ability to cope with diabetes" (Boehnert & Popkin, 1986). Clinical case studies report threats of suicide as well as acting out of self-destructive behavior, such as "forgetting" or deliberately omitting insulin, or deviating from the prescribed diet. For one such patient, repeated omission of insulin served as a means of exercising imagined control over the illness, and was seen as a measure of potential control over the time and place of death. In a study of deliberate self-poisoning among diabetic patients, the majority used a range of nondiabetic drugs; a small majority deliberately overdosed on insulin (Jefferys & Volans, 1983).

One of the fears of diabetes is the possibility of going blind. Should the therapist become aware that eye problems are developing, it is important to get medical advice regarding the prognosis. If blindness appears to be inevitable, the subject of rehabilitation should be introduced so the patient has time to go through the long and tedious process of developing compensatory hearing and tactile abilities. Therapists should not collaborate with the patient's denial. Blindness can result in suicide, particularly with severely depressed patients who have not confronted their problems (Caplan, 1981).

8.4.5. Kidney Disease

Patients with kidney disease must deal with the ramifications of chronic renal failure, hemodialysis, and kidney transplantation. Their ambivalence about life is expressed in both a fear of death and a fear of life. Irreversible kidney failure or end stage renal disease (ESRD) may be caused by a wide variety of conditions, illnesses, or accidents. The two most common causes are inflammation of the capillary loops of the glomeruli of the kidney (called glomerulonephritis, about 25%) and diabetes (about 15%). In the early stages, there may be no overt physical or psychological symptoms. Later, a variety of symptoms develop, referred to as the uremic syndrome. These include insomnia, nausea, vomiting, diarrhea, emotional lability, drowsiness, confusion, fatigue, difficulties in concentration, muscle cramps, seizures, and weight loss (Binik, 1983). Kidney disease usually develops after age 45, and the rate of deterioration is quite variable.

There are a number of stressors involved in ESRD. One is the uncertainty about survival and the rate of development and deterioration, which, as noted, is quite variable. Patients become dependent upon medical staff for treatment of the disease and its complications, and changes in staff or the organization of treatment delivery can result in significant stress. Hemodialysis and peritoneal dialysis involve severe restrictions in diet and fluid intake, as well as in mobility and opportunities for travel. Patients on hemodialysis need to be near hospitals or centers where they receive their treatment. Also, dialysis can be very demanding on time. For example, hemodialysis usually involves three treatment sessions per week, three to five hours each. During this time, the patient's blood is circulated outside the body through an artificial kidney, a very psychologically stressful experience. Although in some cases this can be done at home, the procedure requires adequate facilities and intensive training of those involved. Another form of treatment, peritoneal dialysis, utilizes the patient's peritoneum as an artificial kidney by filling the abdominal cavity with fluid, so that waste products and fluid pass from the blood vessels of the peritoneum into the dialysate fluid by process of diffusion. Treatment may be delivered intermittently (e.g., twice weekly at the hospital for 18 or more hours) or continuously (Continuous Ambulatory Peritoneal Dialysis, CAPD) by means of an indwelling catheter and a bag of dialysate, which needs to be exchanged about four times per day. Each exchange may take between 40 and 60 minutes. Even a kidney transplantation makes extreme demands, often requiring two to three months of hospitalization.

Treatment schedules may conflict with work, resulting in loss of income or job. Some patients may feel generally weak and sickly, while others may suffer from complications such as blood disease, anemia, and muscle cramps. Side effects from medication can be debilitating, and hobbies and social activities may need to be limited or given up entirely for lack of time, energy, and resources.

Despite all these difficulties, recent studies have not shown depression to be as important a factor for ESRD patients as previously thought (Binik, 1983). However, anxiety and suicidal ideation are not uncommon (Livesley, 1981). Although most ESRD patients do not actively take their own lives, passive approaches have been noted, such as withdrawing from dialysis programs, inability or refusal to follow dietary and fluid restrictions, or not taking proper care of the shunt (Abram, 1978). Active approaches have included cutting the shunt, overdosing on medication, or using firearms. In a study of 3478 dialysis patients (Abram, Moore, & Westervelt, 1971), 1 out of 20 ended life through active or passive means: 29 withdrew from the dialysis program, 117 died from the inability or refusal to follow medical regimens, 20 committed suicide. Another 17 attempted suicide but failed.

In a more recent study of 209 patients, 26% died 2.5 to 7.5 years after receiving their first kidney transplantation; of those who died, 8 (15%) committed suicide (Washer, Schroter, Starzl, & Weil, 1983). The authors conclude that many patients on chronic dialysis see successful transplantation as their last hope, and become quite despondent if there is graft failure. Also, the alteration of physical appearance as a consequence of steroid treatment can be unduly upsetting, particularly for the young.

8.4.6. Huntington's Disease

Huntington's disease is a neurological disorder that usually occurs in midlife. It results in progressive involuntary movements and cognitive impairment, which can be preceded or accompanied by emotional disturbance (see discussion in Chapter 3). Research suggests that these patients are at significant risk for suicide, as compared with the general population. In a study of people with Huntington's disease, where the cause of death had been established, those between the ages of 10 and 49 were almost three times as likely to commit suicide as those in the general population of the same age. For patients 50 to 69 years of age, the rate was 23 times as likely (Schoenfeld *et al.*, 1984).

8.4.7. Respiratory Diseases

Chronic obstructive pulmonary disease (COPD) is a term that applies to a group of respiratory disorders, including chronic bronchitis, asthma, and emphysema. A high number of suicides have been reported for this population (Sawyer, Adams, Conway, Reeves & Kvale, 1983). In the study of hospital suicides (Farberow *et al.*, 1971), patients with respiratory diseases accounted for 11.7% of the physically ill patients who committed suicide in the VA hospitals surveyed. Given their number within the hospital population, this was 3.8% more than would have been expected.

COPD is often progressive. When patients first begin treatment, there may be unrealistic expectations that they will eventually be back to normal. Initially they become optimistic, a feeling that is reinforced by increased staff attention. In time, feelings of hopelessness and discouragement develop as they begin to realize that their prognosis for recovery is poor. They also begin to realize that as their condition worsens, they will become more and more dependent upon oxygen equipment and on other people. The loss of hope for relief and the fear of the future can lead to depression and, in some cases, suicide.

Persons with asthma also seem to be at particular risk. A review of hospital charts in Canada revealed that they had a higher incidence of suicidal ideation and suicide attempts than those with COPD (Levitan, 1983). And three times as many persons with asthma actually attempted suicide, as compared with those who only entertained the idea.

8.4.8. Cardiovascular Disease

Feelings of depression, rejection, and abandonment were found to be strong predictors of suicide attempts in hospitalized cardiorespiratory patients (Farberow, McKelligott, Cohen, & Darbonne, 1966). However, in the study of suicides in VA general medical and surgical hospitals (Farberow *et al.*, 1971), patients with circulatory problems accounted for 15.8% of the suicides, which was 1.1% over and above what would have been expected given the proportion they represented in the hospital population.

Levitan (1983) found a relatively high incidence of suicidal ideation and suicide attempts in those with hypertension; however, the attempts were fewer in number than those in the asthmatic group, and sample sizes were small. Dorpat, Anderson, and Ripley (1968) had reported earlier that hypertension headed the list of those with psychosomatic illnesses who attempted suicide, and was third on the list for completed suicides. The depressive effects of the amine-depleting drugs used in the treatment of hypertension have been suggested as factors affecting the high suicide rate for hypertensive patients. However, none of the patients in Levitan's study who exhibited suicidal trends were being treated with such medication.

8.4.9. Spinal Cord Injury

The mortality rate for spinal-cord-injured patients after discharge from the hospital is higher than for the general population. In a Canadian study, suicide was one of the causes of death that increased significantly over a seven-year period; the greatest incidence was noted for the complete quadraplegics, who demonstrated a fourfold growth rate (Geisler, Jousse, Wynne-Jones, & Breithaupt, 1983). Paradoxically, the increase in suicide may be due in part to the improved medical care that enables more of these seriously injured patients to survive.

8.5. STAFF ATTITUDE AND DEATH

Others' attitudes can affect the ability of patients to cope with their suicidal feelings. Looking at the suicide rate on a chronic pulmonary ward, Glickman (cited in Moran, 1985) compared the period when the house staff were unhappy dealing with chronic illnesses with the period when the ward was under the direct care of the senior staff physicians. He found that the suicide rate was significantly lower when the senior physicians were the patients' caretakers.

There is a tendency for staff working with terminally ill patients to avoid the dying patient (e.g., pulmonary disease—Agle & Baum, 1977; cancer—Hansen & McAleer, 1983–1984). This accounts in part for dying patients' reports of feeling emotionally abandoned. On the other hand, studies have shown that if terminal patients find the staff to be understanding, sympathetic, not frightened of death themselves, and not likely to abandon them in the terminal stages, they will be more able to accept the fact of their own termination and to make choices that are more satisfying (Farberow et al., 1963).

The health care professionals' own death anxiety, however, affects their perception and how they treat the dying suicidal patient (Hansen & McAleer, 1983–1984). Professionals with high anxiety regarding death were found to rate the patient as more irrational, and more likely to make a successful suicide attempt than were those with medium and low anxiety. High anxiety professionals also reported that they would employ active prevention strategies, such as involuntary hospitalization. When the professionals find a patient's suicidal thoughts and behaviors personally understandable, maybe even acceptable, a serious dilemma occurs when ethical and legal considerations dictate that they are to act otherwise.

8.6. THE RIGHT TO DIE

Therapists and other health care professionals, by and large, share the societal belief that suicide is generally an act of a mentally disturbed person, and thus an act that should be prevented in the person's best interests. However, in the case of those with cancer or other terminal illness, an exception is sometimes made (Gurrister & Kane, 1978; Hansen & McAleer, 1983–1984).

Suicide may not be viewed so harshly in circumstances where the quality of life is severely compromised, i.e., where the patient is in great pain or is severely disfigured, and cannot recover. As much as 37% of the population, in fact, now consider suicide to be an acceptable alternative to death from serious or terminal illness (Huchcroft, 1984). Associations have sprung up in the United States (e.g., the Hemlock Society) and in Europe championing the right to suicide as an expression of control over one's fate, particularly where painful and terminal illness is involved. Some people make a "living will," specifying while they are still in good health that they do not want exceptional measures taken to preserve life should they become terminally ill.

A national poll conducted in the United States by the Roper Organization in 1986 revealed that 75% of those interviewed believed that a physician should be bound by law to obey a dying patient's living will; 62% believed that physicians should have the right to give lethal medications to dying patients who request them—something that is lawful in The Netherlands following certain criteria (National Hemlock Society, 1986, 1987).

The concept of the "rational suicide" has been evolving and implies no psychiatric disorder (Battin, 1982). The reasoning of the suicidal person is not impaired and the motives seem justifiable, or at least understandable. The dying patient's right to choose a direction that could end life, such as refusing treatment, rests on the assumption of informed consent (Ramsey, 1972; Rodin et al., 1981). In situations involving the termination of life support, therapists may be brought in to evaluate a patient's mental competence, to determine if the patient understands the alternatives and is making a deliberate choice. However, the assumption that the patient understands fully the probable course of the disease, or the treatment choices, alternatives, and consequences, is questionable, even when he or she appears to be in fairly good health. Patients and their families are under much stress, and to a large extent make decisions emotionally, rather than rationally, putting great trust in their physicians (Morrow, Gootnick, & Schmale, 1978). Also, such a decision may be temporally distorted by pain, medication, or metabolic abnormality, and may need to be reassessed periodically. Basically, the question is as much ethical as it is legal and medical, and it is still surrounded by much controversy (S.M. Levy, 1983; Siegel & Tuckel, 1984–1985).

9

Facing Death

9.1. The Dying Patient

Those working with the terminally ill have noted that patients tend to go through certain stages in trying to deal with the monumental awareness of their own death and the pain and suffering that may precede it (e.g., Dilley *et al.*, 1986). One of the earliest and most well-known description of the stages of death and dying is that proposed by Kübler-Ross (1970): denial, anger, bargaining, depression, and acceptance. Not all patients go through all the stages, nor do they necessarily go through them in the same order. And as certain crises or plateaus are reached, certain stages may be repeated. It is useful to keep in mind that these reactions are natural, and that they represent ways of dealing with the shock and overwhelming feelings that emerge.

9.1.1. The Stage of Denial

Years ago it was common for physicians to play into the denial. It was considered giving patients hope, something the physicians felt was necessary for survival. Although one cannot dispute the importance of hope, encouraging patients to remain in the stage of denial is not necessarily the best way to help them prepare emotionally or practically for their departure from life.

There is no clear-cut way of ascertaining when a patient knows he or she is going to die. Even when this is stated directly by a physician, denial and bargaining may still come into play. Related to this is what Weisman and Hackett (1962) have labeled "middle knowledge." This is a state of uncertainty about one's condition and destiny. A slight improvement may be seized upon as a good omen, and there may be a marked change in behavior as the depression lifts. But this state is usually transient. In some cases, patients may deny symptoms, despite the fact that their condition has worsened. However, the denial is not total. But caretakers may feel relieved, leading to a period of mutual avoidance. Clinical evidence suggests, however, that most patients do not deny the eventuality of death but do find it hard to accept that it is coming soon (Plumb & Holland, 1981).

Dr. F had not told Don that he had cancer. Instead he had used the word *tumor*. When Don asked if it were benign or malignant, Dr. F replied that that was not a relevant question, for benign cancers sometimes kill, and malignant cancers are not always life-threatening. Thus, he avoided answering the real question: What is my prognosis? In this case, Dr. F was aware that Don was in the advanced stages of lung cancer and had already informed Don's wife that he had less than a year to live. Don, however, clung to the word *tumor* and used it when describing his condition. Yet he constantly complained to his wife that he felt Dr. F was not answering his questions, that he was trying to hide something from him. Although angry that the physician was being evasive, he was ambivalent about wanting to know. One day after hearing his complaints again, his wife knowingly suggested, "Maybe Dr. F knows something that he is hesitant to tell you. Would you want him to?" Don's eyes widened, he paused, then replied, "It was hard enough for me to get through it the first time [i.e., hearing he had a tumor]; I don't think I could handle it again." The physician had missed his chance to openly talk to Don; now his wife, taking her cues from Don, said no more.

However, a few weeks later his wife inadvertently used the word *cancer*. Don looked up at her in surprise. "Is that what I have?" he asked. She, realizing for the first time that the doctor had purposely been avoiding the use of the word *cancer*, replied, "Oh, I don't know. I thought tumor and cancer were the same thing, but that's just my mistake." Later that evening, she overheard Don talking to a friend on the phone about his "cancer." The next day she told the physician what she had done and he was startled. "Didn't he get angry with you?" Dr. F asked. Don's wife was taken aback. Apparently, the doctor had been interpreting the stage of anger as something unpleasant, something to be avoided.

9.1.2. The Stage of Anger

In Don's case, he never really entered an obvious stage of anger, but his repressed anger broke through periodically. Although he tended to intellectualize and ask a multitude of questions during his medical appointments, at home he ranted and raved about the physicians' evasiveness and attempts to treat him like a child. He also became extremely frustrated and impatient with his own physical weakness and the resulting dependency. He yelled at his wife for not preparing food the way he wanted it. When friends came over to help rearrange the furniture in his room to make it more comfortable for him, he flew into a rage because they took so long to get it done. His wife's best friend, hearing the tirade, asked with wide eyes: "Is he always like this?"

But Don was basically a quiet, kindly man; the anger only came to the surface when he encountered stressful situations. His characteristic way of coping had been through isolation of affect and denial, and these defenses came into play during his illness. In speaking about having cancer, he was able to intellectualize and isolate the affect to give him time to deal with the impact of what he was going through.

9.1.3. The Stage of Bargaining

The bargaining stage is the period of trying to regain some control, to be a participant, and to gain some time. For example, at first the idea of extensive treatment may seem unendurable; in time, however, cooperating with the physician becomes a means of bargaining. "If I'm good and do what they [the authority figures] tell me to do, maybe I will get well, or at least not get any worse."

Don did his share of bargaining. He quit smoking even though he suspected it was too late. He followed the medical routines religiously, and despite his increasing difficulty swallowing, tried to eat healthful foods. Once his wife let him sleep rather than waking him for medication because "he looked so peaceful that I couldn't bring him back to his suffering." But his anger reappeared with a vengeance because she had interfered with his bargaining.

When diseases do not get better, or when they recur, patients often feel betrayed. After all, they did everything they were supposed to.

9.1.4. The Stage of Depression

As an illness progresses, depression sets in. It may be quite severe or an underlying depression that gnaws at the patient. Weisman (1978) has speculated that much of the depression, loneliness, and regression found among terminally ill patients is in response to the professionals' "conspiracy of silence" (p. 187). When confronted with an incurable patient, professionals often respond from their own prejudices and uncertainties, falling back on the typical professional defenses of emotional isolation, standoffishness, and intellectualized professionalism. This stance leaves the patient in an atmosphere of deception, denial, and censorship. Instead of being able to face death with dignity, patients find themselves feeling abandoned and socially isolated.

Don, like many patients, experienced endless sleepless nights, filled with anxiety and depression. His wife would wake up in the middle of the night to find him sitting up in bed, sad and frightened. His thoughts wandered to his parents and brothers, from whom he was estranged. He dreamed of going back to his hometown to make amends (bargaining reappearing to help lift the depression).

Although physicians may ply patients with medication, it is often not effective when thoughts of life and death lie heavy on the patient's mind. Sometimes psychotherapists have had some success in getting the patient to use thought-stopping or relaxation techniques, and individual and family psychodynamic therapy sessions can be useful in reducing tension.

9.1.5. The Stage of Acceptance

Depression begins to lift as the patient enters the stage of acceptance. This is not necessarily a permanent stage, but one that a person goes into and retreats from periodically. During this period, patients allow themselves to be reassured that they do not have to feel in total control, and to recognize that the suffering is about to be over. It is also the period of saying good-bye to important people, but, once done, the farewells permit a relaxation and an acceptance of what is to come. To Weisman (1978, p. 187), death is "a reasonable end stage in the longitudinal process of living, and is not thereby an evil, tragic occasion."

Don entered the stage of acceptance close to the day of his death. He tried desperately to contact old friends, whom he'd refused to see during his illness, practically begging them to come to the hospital to see him. He even called one physician to apologize for the excessive rage he'd poured onto this man. The night he died he found himself slipping into unconsciousness, and would force himself awake, sitting bolt upright in bed. Seeing his wide, terrified eyes, his wife asked him if he were afraid. He nodded yes, listened to her reassuring words, "I'm here with you," and slipped into his last sleep.

9.2. PSYCHOTHERAPY AND THE DYING PATIENT

Psychotherapy with the dying is unique and unlike that with other patients. One of the important distinctions is that time is finite. Shneidman (1978), who has written extensively on the subject, sees the goal of therapy as helping the patient achieve a positive quality of life until the end, including freedom from pain. This involves lending as much stability as possible, and permitting patients to tie up loose ends, i.e., putting their affairs in order, emotionally and practically. When one is working with the dying, certain strategies need to be observed (Shneidman, 1978):

1. Let the patient bring up the subject of death and dying; don't force it. And don't run from the topic or from the patient when the subject does come up. Listen.

2. Be flexible; let the patient set the pace. From one session to the next the patient may move from hope to despair and denial. At one time, the patient may be talking about the vacation she will go on once she gets out of the hospital, and at another time about the grim reality of the present moment. The patient may focus on other comparable periods—that is, other endings or stresses, such as the death of a parent or a child. Sometimes a very ill patient will just lie there, eyes closed, still aware of your presence but too weak or tired to continue talking. Sitting quietly with the patient and periodically saying something related to previous discussions can be reas-

suring. Some patients find relaxation techniques and imagery useful for relieving pain or anxiety.

3. Minimize interpretations of latent content. Comfort and peace are more important at this stage than new insights. There may not be time to work through psychodynamic issues, and the person may be left in a state of agitation. Bear in mind that few patients die with "all their complexes and neuroses completely worked through" (Shneidman, 1978, p. 210).

4. Feel free to be more interactive with the terminally ill than is customary in the treatment of others. This can involve making suggestions, giving advice, interacting with doctors, nurses, and family members, and arranging for social services. Discuss with the patient any practical issues that come up, such as burial arrangements or disposition of belongings. Some of these issues are expressions of a continued wish for control or immortality, but, as mentioned before, it is best not to interpret the latent content.

9.3. THE THERAPIST'S REACTION TO DEATH AND DYING

A close bond can develop with the dying patient, despite the effort to maintain a professional distance. It then becomes particularly difficult when one day the therapist enters the patient's hospital room only to find herself being confused with someone else, or not being recognized at all. The patient's reaction may be the result of heavy doses of medication to control pain or symptoms, a lack of oxygen to the brain, metastasis to the brain, or other organic factors. The sense of loss and impotence on the therapist's part is, however, real. And, as the patient's condition worsens, the therapist can find herself becoming depressed and anxious. Transference and countertransference become intense when working with the terminally ill, and when the patient dies, the therapist may find herself grieving.

When terminally ill patients take their own lives, the therapist's reactions are quite complex. Therapists develop a special relationship with their patients and gain special insight into their suffering, both physical and emotional. On one level, the therapist understands the patient's despair, and privately may even support the drastic action. On another level, a sense of loss and failure is present, along with the expected grief associated with death. Gnawing doubts persist about not having done enough, or not having done the right thing; questions linger about the rightness of having "lied" to the patient, by supporting denial when trying to provide encouragement and hope. Yet on another level, the therapist experiences conflicting feelings of relief. There is relief in knowing that the patient is no longer suffering, but there is guilt over the therapist's personal relief that the emotionally draining work is finally over. On a practical level, there may be fears of lawsuits or negative reactions from colleagues or the medical profession, who, in looking for a place to assign their own feelings of impotence, consider suicide a failure of psychotherapy. And finally, there is the confrontation with one's own vulnerability and mortality, issues that are dealt with at length elsewhere in this book (see Chapter 13).

Sometimes a healthy patient may die unexpectedly from an accident or sudden illness, such as a heart attack. In this case, the therapist has not had time to begin mourning prior to the death, as would be the case when working with someone known to be terminally ill. An unexpected loss can leave the therapist in a state of shock. At first, it may be difficult to react, or to grasp the reality of what has happened. There are memories of the last meeting, feelings of empathy and helplessness, of not having been there to comfort or help the patient at the end, and feelings about work left undone.

When a patient dies, questions arise about whether or not to attend the funeral or to contact the family. Family members, who felt cut out of the therapeutic relationship, may not be open to hearing from the therapist. On the other hand, if no attempt is made to communicate, they may question the therapist's lack of feeling and empathy. Depending upon the therapeutic approach and the patient's and the therapist's previous relationship with the family, the therapist may decide to phone or write a letter of condolence. Rarely do therapists attend a funeral, although the desire to do so may exist. In such cases, the therapist should be aware of the countertransference feelings. Being in touch with the family and attending the funeral, may help the therapist to come to terms with the death; however, such behaviors may go beyond the need to grieve and show empathy. They may come from the therapist's need for recognition and reassurance, to show how important he was to the patient and what a good person he, the therapist, is.

The therapist may be confused about what to do regarding the bill. Feelings of guilt arise about sending the bill when others are grieving. One possibility is to wait a couple of months and send a bill to the estate. A therapist who decided not to bother the family with a bill at such a time was surprised to get an insurance form from the family for claims for reimbursement. Following the death of a patient, it is helpful for a therapist to have good support systems, and to seek out a colleague or supervisor to assist in dealing with the feelings and issues raised.

9.4. The Hospice Movement

When discussing the care of the terminally ill, it is necessary to consider the hospice movement. Having developed in Europe, particularly in England, the idea has been spreading in the United States, where the first hospice was started in 1974. Basically, the hospice concept refers to a system of medical care than emphasizes palliation and psychosocial support for terminally ill patients and their families (Greer et al., 1986). Hospices provide a supportive environment for the terminally ill at home or in special "home-like" settings in which there is a minimum of professional intervention. In the United States, hospices are either hospital-based or home care. Most of the patients involved have diagnoses of cancer, and the majority are in a home care situation.

In the early 1980s a National Hospice Study was conducted to evaluate the impact of hospice care on the patients' quality of life (Greer & Mor, 1986). Because of the emphasis on home care in the United States, there was some concern that those in home care settings would suffer because they would not have access to pain control and other medical interventions that could alleviate unpleasant symptoms.

The results of the study suggest that the terminally ill patients and their families appear to fare equally well when patients are in hospices or in conventional settings (Aiken, 1986). However, differences were noted. The hospices do provide a different constellation of services: less diagnostic testing, less aggressive antitumor therapy in the terminal period, and more social services, including counseling. Hospitals with inpatient hospice units appear to provide better pain control, possibly as a result of more liberal use of analgesics, and their patients had fewer symptoms, such as nausea, than those in the conventional settings or home care hospices (Aiken, 1986). More research is needed to better understand the interaction of factors that provide the best emotional atmosphere and treatment.

10

Facing Life

10.1. THE STRENGTHENED BODY

People assume that working with physically ill patients must be morbid. "Isn't it depressing?" is a question often asked. Yet most of the work, unless one specializes in terminal illness, is with those who need help in facing life. Because of advances in detection as well as treatment, many who previously would have died now have their illnesses cured or arrested (Cella & Tross, 1986; Clark, Hailstone, & Slade, 1979; Stone, 1975). For example, the five-year survival rate for all sites of cancer combined is more than 50% (National Cancer Institute, 1984). And recurrence is rare after five years for many types of cancer, including Hodgkin's disease and testicular, endometrial, and cervical cancer.

Although a significant number of cancer patients are reaching the 5-year survival rate, many still face the possibility of recurrence 15 to 20 years later (Li, Cassady, & Jaffe, 1975). And some of the aggressive therapies leave the patient at significant risk for later physical complications (Cella & Tross, 1986). It appears that after the acute stages of the illness have passed, the patient's psychosocial adjustment can become as important to the illness as the person's physical state (Belgrave & Washington, 1986; Derogatis, 1986).

10.2. THE STRENGTHENED EGO

Despite impairments in physical abilities and reductions in quality of life, seriously ill patients have been found to make reasonably satisfactory adjustments to their conditions (Heinrich & Schag, 1985a). Worden and Sobel (1978), in a study of newly diagnosed cancer patients, found that good ego strength is associated with fewer physical symptoms. This raises the question: Does ego strength affect the course of the disease, or is it simply a reflection of the person's medical condition?

Patients survive with greater and lesser degrees of disability, which make demands on the person's psychological integrity and social support systems. And many patients must live with psychological stresses related to the unknown course of their illness. Time seems to be a positive factor in helping people adjust to serious illness (Cassileth *et al.*, 1984; Cella & Tross, 1986; Clark *et al.*, 1979). Research conducted with those suffering from arthritis, diabetes, cancer, renal disease, and dermatological disorders reveals that those recently diagnosed exhibit more anxiety, depression, and feelings of loss of control than do those who have lived with their illness for more than four months. And patients whose active treatment is behind them feel psychologically stronger than those currently undergoing treatment, particularly treatment that is physically demanding. Thus, it appears that, over time, patients gain greater emotional distance from the acute traumas associated with the illness.

10.3. POSITIVE EMOTIONS

When positive emotions are expressed by those who are seriously ill, others often react with surprise and interpret the unexpected positive feelings as denial and a distortion of the "real," more appropriate feelings. Yet there is a growing body of evidence revealing that seriously ill patients do have positive emotions and experiences, including feelings of competence, satisfying interpersonal relationships, and less depression than expected (Bukberg *et al.*, 1984; Trillin, 1981; Viney, 1986).

Some studies suggest that for many patients quality of life is very similar to that of the general population (Binik, 1983; Heinrich & Schag, 1985a). One woman, severely disabled from an automobile accident, discovered to her own surprise that she felt stronger than before, and that she liked herself better. "I never had much confidence in myself. I never thought I could do all of the things I am doing now," she confided, referring to the way she had organized her life and continued despite her disabilities.

10.3.1. Measuring Adjustment to Illness

Various scales have been devised to measure adjustment to medical illness. One is the Psychosocial Adjustment to Illness Scale (PAIS, or PAIS-SR for the self-report form), developed by Derogatis (1986). This scale has loadings on six factors: social environment, vocational environment, sexual relationships, health care orientation, extended family relationships, and psychological distress (see Table 1). Data are being gathered on six normative medical samples: lung cancer, renal dialysis, acute burn, essential hypertension, cardiac disease, and mixed cancer. The evidence collected thus far suggests that this instrument will be useful in differentiating between those who are adjusting well and those who are not.

TABLE 1. Psychological Adjustment Scale (PAIS-SR): Sample Questions[a]

I. Social environment: "Have you maintained your interests in social activities since your illness (e.g., social clubs, church groups, going to the movies)?"

II. Vocational environment: "Is your work as important to you now as it was before your illness?"

III. Sexual relationships: "When some people become ill, they report a loss of interest in sex; have you experienced a reduction of sexual interest associated with your illness?"

IV. Health care orientation: "Describe for me your general attitude and approach to taking care of your health."

V. Extended family relationships: "Do you normally depend on members of your extended family for physical or financial assistance? Has this changed at all since your illness?"

VI. Psychological distress: "Have you been feeling less adequate, helpless, or down on yourself since your illness?"

---

[a]Source: From Derogatis (1986).

10.3.2. Locus of Control

Feelings of personal control are related to successful adaptation to severe and chronic illness (Williams & Stout, 1985). Rotter's (1966) constructs of internal and external locus of control (LOC) have been applied to understanding the way people react to illness and the accompanying state of powerlessness (e.g., Belgrave & Washington, 1986; Schroeder & Miller, 1983). Those with external LOC attribute success and failure to fate or to powerful others, and believe that what one does matters little. Internals, on the other hand, are more likely to see rewards and punishments occurring as a result of their own behavior.

In a study of patients with peripheral vascular disease, Schroeder and Miller (1983) found that externals were more likely to use denial, express feelings of guilt, and be passive regarding their condition. Internals, on the other hand, actively looked for ways to be involved in the decisions concerning their treatment and attempted to develop skills needed for self-care. In a study of patients with tuberculosis, Seeman and Evans (1962) found that internals were more likely to seek out information about their disease than were externals.

Most studies conclude that those with internal locus of control are better adjusted, with some suggesting that patients be trained to be more assertive and interactive in their care (Brooks and Richardson, 1980; Schuler, 1982; Wolpe, 1980). The research, however, is sparse and not consistent in its findings regarding which style is the most beneficial to patients' health in the long run. A study of diabetics (Lowery & DuCette, 1976) revealed the unexpected result that patients with an external LOC showed a significant decrease in frequency of health-related problems over time, whereas no such decrease occurred for the internals. The authors suggest that the willingness of the externals to leave control in the hands of others and to follow the orders of their physicians may have contributed to their better health. External LOC could be preferable for managing illnesses such as diabetes, where dietary restrictions and other life-style and medical routines need to be followed closely. However, more research is needed to see which LOC is most effective for dealing with other diagnoses.

10.4. FACING THE FUTURE: THE RETURN TO WORK

Returning to work can be fraught with anxiety. Certain illnesses, if they change people's appearance, make it difficult for them to deal with the public, because of their own personal discomfort as well as the public's reactions. Examples of physical changes are facial disfigurement resulting from accident, surgery, or facial tumors; severe loss of weight; and ambulatory problems.

Patients may fear that they no longer can perform as they once did, that they lack stamina or the physical wherewithal. If the condition is chronic or has the possibility of recurring, the patient may struggle with the questions of "if" and "when" to tell a prospective employer. Afraid of discrimination, many conceal their disorders, if they can, for fear of not getting a job, or being fired from one they already have. This has added risks, however, for if there is an attack or recurrence of symptoms on the job, others may not be prepared to help. There is also the psychological stress of having to keep a feared secret and the fear of being found out.

One of the realities, however, is that there is still some discrimination in the work force directed toward those who have had a serious illness or disability (Colorez & Geist, 1987; Freidenbergs et al., 1981–1982; Kokaska & Maslow, 1986; Perry & Apostal, 1986). This has been especially true for those with illnesses such as cancer, epilepsy, heart disease, renal disease, diabetes, and hypertension.

Yet a nationwide survey (ICD, 1987) of managers revealed that employers described disabled employees as hardworking, reliable, and productive. In addition, the cost of employing the disabled was not seen as a significant barrier. Still, employers give hiring the disabled a lower priority than hiring people from minority groups or the elderly. Subsequently, two-thirds of the disabled persons between 16 and 64 are not working, even though two-thirds of them would like to work (ICD, 1986).

Those who have been ill or are physically disabled are discriminated against, not only because of rationalizations related to economic factors (i.e., "Will they be able to do the job?") but because many people feel uncomfortable in the presence of the disability and illness (i.e., "It will upset my customers"). There are also demographic factors that affect a person's return to work, as well. One is socioeconomic (SES). Decreased strength and energy has a greater effect on those in the lower SES, who generally work at more manual occupations as compared with professional and business positions. Also, their motivation for returning may not be great since they may not be as highly compensated or as emotionally invested in their work. Gender also plays a role. A housewife may be able to return to household work more easily than a man can return to his place of employment. This is becoming less true as more and more women are entering the work force. Also, certain responsibilities in maintaining a house require strength and stamina, which an ill spouse may no longer have.

Disabled people who are working report greater satisfaction with life than do nonworking disabled persons. They are less likely to consider themselves disabled or to feel that their disability has prevented them from reaching their full potential as individuals (ICD, 1986). Setting unrealistic goals is not advisable, but patients do need to be encouraged to try to return to their former occupations, if at all feasible. At certain stages of recuperation, for example, the patient may be able to do work at home, particularly if computers and telephones can be utilized.

Molly, a woman who was now homebound and in a wheelchair, struggled with the question of whether to tell the employer of her illness and disability. Through former colleagues, she had been given a project that could be done at home. Although she had never met the employer and could conduct her business by letter and phone, she feared the consequences should the employer find out she was disabled. The disability was not expected to affect the outcome of her performance, although she might be slower than before. She also feared she might develop some physical complications and have to abort the project.

Through psychotherapy Molly came to realize that she indeed had budgeted sufficient time for the project, that becoming ill again was not highly probable and could happen to an able-bodied person, and that the assistant she was going to hire could carry much of the work load should she be temporarily incapacitated. Basically, what needed to be worked through were issues related to her poor self-image; these involved performance anxiety that predated her illness, and the yet-to-be-tested assumptions about others' possible negative reactions to her disability.

Even if Molly's employer had found out about her disability, the results might not have been as negative as she feared. As it turned out, the actual problems were not as critical as anticipated. And had he known, the employer might have been more accepting than expected. Efforts have been made over the years to prevent the medically ill from job discrimination (e.g., Stone, 1975; Wheatley, Cunnick, Wright, & van Keuren, 1974). The laws, however, affect larger companies and those under governmental contracts. For some, insurance benefits for continuation of income at times of disability have become more generous. In many large companies, employees with certain number of months of service are entitled to income benefits during illness, depending upon their length of service. Still there are those who face financial hardship and worry about reentry into the job market.

Leonard, a clothing salesman, had been working for a clothing manufacturer for 35 years. On his 65th birthday, just when he was considering cutting back his hours and "enjoying his life," he was diagnosed as having prostate cancer. The clothing company, although fairly large, was a family-run firm, with modest health and disability benefits. Leonard had stopped going to work because of the radiation and chemotherapy treatments and his severe reaction to them. Although the company kept him on their books for the health coverage, they did not pay him a salary. They also said they could not guarantee him his job if he stayed out of work too long. Tired, weak, and demoralized, Leonard felt as though he had been betrayed by those he had worked for most of his adult life. He found himself applying for social security benefits and what he called "welfare." For him it was hard to think of a future.

Matt, a 59-year-old drug salesman, was laid off from his company after 40 years of service, when the company was taken over by another firm. During this period of unemployment he was diagnosed as having a malignant melanoma on his leg. He became terribly depressed because he now had to deal with many losses at one time: the loss of his job, the loss of mobility from the extensive incision on his leg, and the possible loss of his life from the melanoma. He felt totally useless and spent most of his time obsessing about his leg. After several months, he began working with the counselors at a vocational guidance clinic, where they helped him in his job search. He eventually did find work, but not at his previous level.

These examples show that anguish is a natural part of the process of facing life again. The patients' perception of themselves as diminished can be a reflection of the way society sees them. Although it may be realistic in some cases that patients cannot do what they once did, the patients and society often operate from old prejudices, misinformation, and unfounded fear. Once patients regain strength and develop new conceptions of themselves, they often are able to reenter life, surprising themselves and others with how much they can accomplish and how good they feel.

III

Practical and Philosophical Considerations: The Therapist's Role

11

Interpersonal/Professional Concerns

11.1. REFERRALS FROM PHYSICIANS

Physical and psychological problems frequently occur at the same time, and a closer working relationship between physicians and therapists is needed to improve clinical care. Many physicians assume that the patients' emotional turmoil, though painful, is simply part of the process. This attitude was illustrated by one surgeon who, when commenting on his work with facially disfigured patients, sighed: "God help them. They somehow manage." It apparently did not occur to him that someone other than God could help ease their psychological pain.

Compounding the problem is the fact that physicians frequently do not recognize psychiatric illness in their medical patients (Schwab, 1982), or, conversely, they assign psychological explanations to emotional reactions and disturbing behaviors that are primarily a function of the illness and its treatment (Hayes, Butler, & Martin, 1986). When physicians do refer, it may be because they have had experience with serious illness in their personal lives (Taylor & Chrisler, 1988).

In most cases, however, physicians attempt to deal with psychological difficulties, rather than referring patients for professional psychological help (Fink & Shapiro, 1966). Many are skeptical of psychotherapy. Others underestimate or deny the severity of the underlying problems, or overestimate their own ability to be of help.

A wide disparity exists between the prevalence of mental disorders among medical and surgical patients and the number of psychiatric referrals (Hertz, Greenberg, & Baredes, 1984). In a study of cancer patients, for example, Levine, Silverfarb, and Lipowski (1978) found that fewer patients were referred for psychological consultation than would be expected from the prevalence of mental disorders in the general population. In addition to the psychological complications inherent in having a physical illness, many patients seen by physicians, such as those with self-inflicted injuries, somatoform disorders, or prior psychiatric illness, have emotional problems that would be amenable to psychological intervention.

Not referring patients may actually do a disservice. Studies (Rosen & Wiens, 1979) have shown that referral for psychological treatment, even on a short-term basis, can have an impact on medical care, such as reducing the eventual number of actual medical visits needed. One reason for this impact may be that patients need to be reassured that some of the feelings they have are related to emotional rather than medical causes. They may also need to be reassured that their concerns are being taken seriously, that their fears and feelings are natural or at least understandable, given their history and the ordeal that they are going through.

At times when physicians do make referrals for psychotherapy, they may expect results too soon, and become angry that the patient "has not been cured yet." Reactions may range from the physician's ignoring the therapist's input, to attempting to engage another mental health professional who promises results, to rapidly changing the protocol expected of the patient without notifying or consulting with the treating psychotherapist. Borderline patients, in particular, may relish this conflict, since they become the center of attention and do not have to focus on important issues of denial and possible physical complications.

11.1.1. Hospital Consultations

Therapists may get a referral to do a psychological consultation or evaluation of a new patient who is hospitalized for medical reasons. Such referrals may be initiated by physicians or the family. Although the therapists may see themselves as coming to lend emotional support to the patient, they may not be greeted warmly. Patients may feel a great deal of apprehension and may question the purpose of the consultation. They may not have been informed about the visit or, if told, not given sufficient information. Sometimes physicians are not comfortable in their own minds about psychotherapy, and they may minimize the psychiatric referral by casually mentioning, "Pat Brown will stop by to see you about your depression," with no explanation of Pat Brown's professional role. One patient, upon learning that the person who just walked into the room was a psychologist, replied apprehensively, "I know why you are here. They sent you to break the bad news to me." Another patient felt that the physician had given up on him, and another was skeptical about the stated supportive nature of the referral, wondering if the referring physician thought he might be crazy.

The role a therapist can play in a hospital setting depends upon the therapist's qualifications, status in terms of the hospital (on staff or not), the hospital regulations, and the state regulations. If therapists are on staff or have hospital privileges, they may be able to see patients regularly. If not, special permission may be needed to make professional visits in the hospital (American Psychological Association, 1985).

11.2. REFERRALS TO PHYSICIANS

Therapists need to be alert to the possibility of the development of a physical illness in their private patients (Silverman, 1985). Ruling out the underlying basis of physical complaints, however, becomes difficult, particularly when the patient has a history of hypochondriasis.

Getting a complaining patient to see a physician can be a problem, particularly if the therapist's traditional role has been nondirective. Some patients' denial may not let them bring up concerns about their health for some time, and after mentioning these concerns, they may ignore or minimize them in subsequent sessions. If a serious illness is suspected, therapists may need to introduce the subject again, stepping out of the nondirective role to urge the patients to have an examination. It is best to help patients mobilize their resources to find their own physician, if they don't have one. Only if a patient is unable to do so, for special reasons, or if the therapist is aware of a physician with a unique, required specialty, should a recommendation be made. Recommending a specific physician, however, can be fraught with problems, since the patient may later blame the therapist if there are any difficulties during treatment.

Afterwards, should the therapist wish to speak to the physician to keep abreast of the patient's condition, it is best to obtain approval from the patient. Have the patient notify her physician that she is involved in therapy, and that the therapist may be calling. If the approval is given in writing, a copy can be sent to the physician along with a letter of introduction. Less formal arrangements are often made when the therapist is personally known to the physician, but permission for interchange should be discussed with the patient. If such permission isn't obtained, patients can become quite upset when the physician mentions something that could only have come from the therapist. Even with permission, the therapist must be discreet about how much to say, respecting the patient's confidentiality. Basically, the physician needs to know how the patient is holding up. Suggestions about how much information the patient wants and can handle about the illness and treatment is also useful. Unusual situations in the patient's life that may affect treatment can also be discussed. If the patient has a personality disorder that may cause difficulty with the medical personnel, or is severely emotionally disturbed or potentially suicidal, this would need to be discussed with the physician.

One difficulty is that some physicians become curious about a patient's personal life, and may ask questions that most therapists feel are beyond what is needed for proper medical care (e.g., "Why has Ms. Wilson never married?"). Therapists should gently explain to physicians that they are not free to discuss such issues but certainly will keep the physicians apprised should any patients be under undue emotional stress that might interfere with their treatment.

Once patients begin seeing a physician, they may understandably experience mounting anxiety as a hospital stay or important medical appointment approaches. Therapists should make note of such important dates, since they often underlie mounting anxiety, disorganization, and acting-out.

11.3. PRACTICAL ISSUES: THE PRIVATE PATIENT

A sick patient represents a loss of income, which can be of particular concern to those who are in the early stages of establishing a practice. Patients miss sessions or, when they do come, may not be able to afford the regular fee because of the newly acquired and substantial medical expenses.

Whether or not to charge for home or hospital visits when the patient is seriously ill can become an issue. One way to handle the dilemma of continuity of care is to visit the patient once or twice at the hospital or at home on a no-fee basis. Then if the patient can afford to pay for sessions, regular appointments can be set up, if desired. It should be borne in mind, however, that home and hospital visits have other implications for therapy. The therapist enters into a part of the patient's life heretofore unknown. Patients may have some reservations about wanting the therapist to see how they live, or to encounter family members whom the therapist may not have met.

If the sick patient can no longer afford psychotherapy but wants to continue, the therapist needs to consider the implications of seeing the patient on a no-fee basis. If this is not feasible or desirable, the therapist may help the patient find alternative psychological care, such as making arrangements for Social Service to see the patient in the hospital, or for a visiting counselor from a social service agency (e.g., Cancer Care) to see the patient at home. Another alternative is to arrange for telephone sessions, if the convalescence is to be long term and the patient desires to continue in therapy. (See Chapter 13 for a discussion of other practical issues that arise when the therapist becomes ill.)

12

Knowing and Not Knowing

12.1. TO TELL OR NOT TO TELL

In the legal and medical climate of today, patients are able to demand and expect as much information about their condition as is available. Whereas, in the past, secrecy and deception predominated (Radovsky, 1985), with the advent of more effective treatments, a more relaxed attitude about sharing information is evolving (Koocher, 1986).

In a survey of 699 physicians in the United States, 98% of the 264 who responded said their usual policy was to inform cancer patients of their diagnosis, and 69% either never or very rarely deviated from that policy (Novack et al., 1979). These results stand in marked contrast to those of an almost identical study reported 18 years earlier, in which 90% generally did not inform cancer patients (Oken, 1961). The findings are typical of their time, for up until the middle of the 20th century, the word *cancer* was rarely spoken above a whisper.

Keeping the dreaded information from patients was a way of not taking away hope, something considered necessary for survival and a means of minimizing "unnecessary anxiety." Today, having information is considered less anxiety-producing, because it allows patients to feel they have regained some control by participating in decisions that affect their own care (Krantz & Deckel, 1983).

The open approach to giving information was supported by the results of a study of childhood cancer survivors (Slavin, O'Malley, Koocher, & Foster, 1981). Although telling patients their diagnosis was against the medical advice at the time, those who had been told early in the course of treatment grew up to be better adjusted than those from whom such information had been deliberately withheld. Other studies have supported this approach, suggesting that surviving patients and bereaved family members are better able to cope when communication is more open (Rando, 1983; Spinetta, Swarmer, & Sheposh, 1981).

N.B. Levy (1984), in his work with dialysis patients, recommends informing patients about the possible physical, psychological, and social complications of their treatment. In light of his clinical experience, he feels that if patients are told that depression is likely to accompany the illness and treatment, then they will be more able to deal with it in the long run.

Patients themselves have reported wanting more detailed information about their diagnosis, including the course and treatment of the disease. This is not to say that learning of a dreaded diagnosis is not upsetting. In Denmark (Henriques, Stadil, & Baden, 1980) cancer patients felt strongly that patients should be informed of their diagnosis, even though in the days following disclosure 52% suffered from insomnia and anxiety. None, however, had severe psychiatric reactions. Apparently, many patients would rather deal with the reactions to the knowledge than with the upset created by their own suspicions and fears of the unknown. And, having the opportunity to deal with the knowledge and reaching the stage of acceptance, the majority of patients do not feel stigmatized by their diagnosis, but in fact share this information with family and friends (Cassileth, Zupkis, Sutton-Smith, & March, 1980).

12.1.1. Death and Knowing

Conveying information about imminent death, as compared with a serious illness, raises its own set of issues. Some patients may be aware that they are dying even if not told so directly (Poulton & Powell-Butdorf, 1986). They pick it up from their own bodily cues and the nonverbal behavior of others, who may act with quiet alarm, withdraw, or take an artificial, formal approach toward them.

In reviewing the literature on death and dying, Garfield (1978) and Sobel (1981) conclude that people say they want to know their prognosis. Studies suggest than an open awareness is often more beneficial for patients and their families than mutual pretense (S.M. Levy, 1983). It was interesting to note that in one study, more people felt that they themselves would want to be told if they were dying than felt that others like themselves should be told, and it was generally agreed that the physician should do the telling (Kalish & Reynolds, 1976). It should be noted, however, that many of the studies about knowing or not knowing involve healthy patients. Healthy people may say it is best to know, but this feeling may change when they are really ill.

When prolonged suffering is involved, patients may choose death. In a study of burn patients, 87% of those who were told that the probability of their surviving was poor rejected heroic measures (Imbus & Zawacki, 1977). In the case of dialysis patients, it has been suggested (e.g., Rodin *et al.*, 1981) that these patients be allowed to decide under what circumstances they might want their own treatment discontinued. Such decisions could be reviewed periodically; this would give physicians some direction when patients are no longer mentally able to make informed choices.

12.2. Making the "Right Decision"

In wanting to know their prognosis and in making informed decisions about their treatment, patients may ask for statistical data, such as, "What is the probability that I am going to survive if I opt for this treatment?" Their eventual choices are often dependent upon the way in which the answer to the question is phrased (Kahneman & Tversky, 1984; Tversky & Kahneman, 1981). Although the end result may be the same, whether it is perceived as something to be gained or lost affects the decision. Also, whether an outcome is certain or only probable is another influencing factor. Generally, there is a preference for a sure thing rather than a gamble, even though a successful gamble may have more positive effects.

McNeil, Pauker, Sox, and Tversky (1982) devised an interesting study to analyze how people process and interpret information that is presented statistically. The study focused on operable lung cancer and asked medical patients to choose between two possible treatments: surgery and radiation therapy. Although a number of variables were investigated, only the effects of the "framing" of the information will be discussed here.

Half the subjects received the information in terms of the probability of dying, the other half in terms of the probability of living. The outcomes in each presentation, however, were statistically equal.

For example: "Of 100 people having surgery, 10 will die during treatment, 32 will have died by one year, and 66 will have died by five years. Of 100 people having radiation therapy, none will die during treatment, 23 will die by one year, and 78 will die by five years. Which treatment would you prefer?"

Or: "Of 100 people having surgery, 90 will be alive following treatment, 68 will be alive at the end of one year, and 34 will be alive in five years. Of 100 people having radiation therapy, all 100 will be alive immediately after treatment, 77 will be alive at the end of one year, and 23 will be alive in five years. Which treatment would you prefer?"

The results revealed that the framing of the expected outcomes in terms of probability of living rather than the probability of dying had a substantial effect on people's preferences. Although surgery was the preferred treatment following both presentations, it was much more attractive when data were presented in terms of survival rather than in terms of death, despite the fact that in the long run the outcomes were the same. Even a small risk of dying immediately as a result of an operation must have seemed ominous to many when compared with no deaths immediately after radiation therapy. It was interesting to note that physicians who were also given these choices expressed the same preferences (i.e., showed the same biases) as the patients. This has important implications, since physicians are supposed to be experienced in reading statistical presentations, and they make judgments about treatment plans on the basis of their interpretations. The study raises serious questions about patients' informed participation in their treatment, for the way in which physicians choose to present data can have a significant effect on patients' eventual decisions.

12.3. Issues Involved in Communication

Although patients have direct experience with their illness, they do not necessarily have a greater fund of knowledge about their disease than healthy people (Heinrich & Schag, 1985a). And data suggest that many patients are hesitant to approach physicians or other medical personnel with their complaints or needs for additional information. They may be reluctant because they have no questions to ask, they are fearful of hearing certain answers, or they are discouraged from asking questions by physicians who are defensive and not supportive. Even when informed, patients frequently do not understand the nature or extent of the treatment planned (Isler, 1971; Mitchell & Glicksman, 1977; Peck & Roland, 1977; Taylor, Lichtman, & Wood, 1984). Several repetitions in various forms may be required before a patient is able to comprehend and recall what has been said (Isler, 1971; Rotman, Rogow, DeLeon, & Heskel, 1977). For some, not knowing or not remembering information may serve an adaptive purpose, allowing them to focus on issues that are not disease-related and to get on with their daily living. Thompson (1981) supports this idea and favors withholding information, particularly when patients are trying to deal with the aversive aspects of their illness that are not under their control.

The stage of the illness is important in determining how much information to give (Cox *et al.*, 1986). During the initial stage, the patient and the patient's family may be dealing with the traumatic implications of illness. This is particularly true if it is a lifelong chronic disease, such as diabetes, or a life-threatening one, such as cancer. In the early stages, they may be more receptive to less complex information that includes the basic survival data. Later on they can deal with the more complex explanations about the disease and its treatment.

The literature on the effects of knowing and not knowing, however, is mixed. In a study by Bean, Cooper, Alpert, and Kipnis (1980), 33 chemotherapy patients were interviewed to determine the extent to which they asked questions or sought information. The results showed that the majority (89%) felt they had received sufficient information. For some reason, the authors interpreted this as a notable lack of interest in obtaining further information, rather than an example of good communication. Messerli, Garamendi, and Romano (1980), however, found that the majority of mastectomy patients in their study reported having unanswered questions. Of those who had had operations in the past five years, 47% said they did not know what questions to ask, and 28% reported being too upset to ask anything.

In an extensive study of doctor–patient communication (Waitzkin, 1984, 1985, 1986), patients expressed a strong desire to be informed and felt that information could be helpful to them. However, 65% of the doctors underestimated the patients' desire for information. They also overestimated the amount of actual time they spent with the patients. In an average encounter of about 20 minutes, the doctors spent a little over 1 minute giving information, although they themselves thought that they spent half their time with the patient providing information.

Another significant finding was that physicians tended to initiate questions much more than patients (80–90% of the time), and male physicians interrupted patients more than the patients interrupted the physicians. (Women patients were interrupted more than male patients, but women patients also asked more questions than did male patients.) The physician interruptions may reflect in part their drive to be thorough and efficient, owing to time constraints, but such behavior also interferes with their sensitivity to patient needs and creates dissatisfaction with medical care.

Other studies lend support to the contention that physicians are not good listeners (cited in Studies Show There's Room for Improvement, 1986). In one such study conducted at Wayne State University, doctors interrupted patients after only 18 seconds, on the average. Patients usually have from one to five issues that they want to talk about, but only 23% of the patients said they were able to complete their opening statement. And many never got to all their symptoms because of the interruptions. In another survey conducted by the American Medical Association, more than two-thirds of the respondents stated that doctors do not involve patients enough in treatment decisions, and 65% said that physicians do not spend enough time with patients. These beliefs are among the major reasons that patients change doctors, according to a Harris poll.

12.4. Fear of Knowing and Avoidance of Medical Treatment

A therapist may be asked by a physician, "Why did Mr. Smith take so long to come for an examination?" The answer is often tied into the patient's characteristic ways of handling crisis, which can include denial and avoidance. There may also be historical reasons, such as memories of parents' suffering and death, or family and financial pressures. The following case describes an interplay of factors that resulted in the delay in treating a serious, life-threatening illness.

Jill, a 30-year-old woman, was pregnant with her second child when her physician noticed a suspicious lesion on her belly. The physician wanted to remove the brown spot immediately; however, Jill was afraid to have the excision because it was so close to the fetus. Since Jill's father had had innumerable skin cancers removed over the years, she was not concerned. After all, she told herself, given her father's experience, "Carcinomas are not life-threatening." Her physician went along with her delay, making her promise that she would have the lesion removed immediately after delivery. According to Jill, the physician never mentioned that he suspected the lesion was melanoma. But as she was to explain later, it would have made no difference to her, since she had never heard of (malignant) melanoma.

Four weeks before her delivery, Jill's husband, Sam, had a heart attack. He was only 32, but unbeknownst to him he had congenital heart disease. To add to their fright, both of Sam's parents had died before age 40 of complications from diabetes. The baby was born at the end of March, Sam was recovering from his heart attack, but Jill then developed a serious breast infection. Needless to say, it was months before she went to a dermatologist to remove the little brown spot. Following the biopsy, he informed her that the diagnosis was melanoma. Melanoma, carcinoma, they all sounded the same to her. Jill went home, still her happy self. She called her father on the phone: "What were those spots you had taken off?" she asked. "Melanoma?" "Heavens, no!" he exclaimed. "That's what kills you." And that was how Jill finally learned the seriousness of her condition.

There is no doubt that a huge amount of denial was operating here, as was ignorance about the disease, and a preoccupation with other crises and events in her life. It is quite possible that somewhere along the line one of the physicians did explain to Jill the nature of her condition, but she was unable to absorb the significance of it given the other stresses with which she was coping. Jill's main concern now was that she not be separated from her baby for the melanoma operation because she was nursing. She continued to believe that she was disease-free, although the extent of the disease had yet to be determined.

Knowing can be experienced as threatening in itself. The fear of the diagnosis and treatment can strongly influence the decision not to go to the doctor. Yet with some illnesses, the loss of time can be dangerous, giving the disease time to progress. The delay may in effect cause the feared extensive treatment, the feared pain, the feared disfigurement. Although this is known intellectually by most people, putting off going to the doctor is a common occurrence. "Maybe it's in my mind." "Maybe it will go away." "I'll go to the doctor later when I have more time." In a study of the reasons for avoiding physicians, the five most important factors were the following (Shontz, 1972):

1. Distrust of the physician's competence or skill.
2. Fear of pain and discomfort from medical procedures.
3. Personal dislike of the physician.
4. Wish to avoid the expense of medical treatment.
5. Fear of finding out that one has a serious, perhaps fatal, illness.

Embarrassment is another factor that sometimes plays a role in the procrastination. Patients may fear that the doctor will find out that they are not really ill, and will consider them hypochondriacal and a waste of time.

12.5. Individual Differences

Recent research suggests that individuals differ in their capability and need for self-care and information, and that the best approach may come from matching individual patients to particular strategies (Krantz, Baum, & Wideman, 1980; Krantz & Deckel, 1983). For example, older patients tend to prefer the more traditional and passive role, while younger patients want a greater degree of participation in choices regarding their treatment (Cassileth *et al.*, 1980). Yet too many choices and too much information can be anxiety-producing (Miller, 1981).

In a review of the literature, Miller (1981) found that some people prefer to be informed about the timing and the nature of an aversive event, while others prefer to be distracted from knowing, if the information would be experienced as threatening. Furthermore, patients designated as "deniers" or "avoiders" revealed a slower recovery rate following preoperative preparation, which included giving information regarding the upcoming procedure (Rogers & Reich, 1986). Such patients increase their use of pain medication (Andrew, 1970) and report increased physiological evidence of stress (Shipley, Butt, Horowitz, & Farbry, 1978).

Miller and Mangan (1983) designed a study to tease out differences in coping strategies and the ability to tolerate information. The subjects were gynecological patients about to undergo a colposcopy, i.e., the use of a low-powered microscope to examine the cervix and vagina for abnormal (cancer) cells. Although the procedure is considered medically benign, it could be perceived as invasive and threatening. The patients were divided into two groups on the basis of a self-report scale: information seekers (monitors) and information avoiders (blunters). The results favored matching the amount of information to the patients' preferred coping style. The effect was most notable in the period following the physical examination, where a significant reduction in anxiety (e.g., pulse rate) was exhibited by the blunters, who had been given only minimal information, and the monitors, who had been provided with detailed information. Blunters in general showed fewer signs of stress than did the monitors, revealing that, at least for some, avoidance and denial may be healthy adaptive mechanisms.

This study suggests that listening to patient request for information is a good guide. Those who feel they need it and want it are probably monitors, and therefore would find it helpful. When denied such information, they may become quite anxious and depressed. Those who do not want to know survive well with their avoidance (although it is recognized that they need minimal information to take care of themselves). They are, however, more willing to turn everything over to their physician's care, and may become upset if given too much information.

Complicating the understanding of patients' ability to cope with information is the finding that social class and sex differences play a role in the way people express their need for information. Working-class patients and men are less likely to verbally request information, yet their reported desire for information is equal to the desires of those who initiate discussions and ask questions. Thus, physicians often misperceive the patients' desire to be informed (Waitzkin, 1984, 1985, 1986).

Basically, communication between physician and patient is important because it affects the quality of health care. If patients are not informed, they cannot later give adequate medical histories and may not properly comply with doctors' instructions, or they may delay in reporting significant symptoms and getting appropriate care.

13

Implications of the Therapist's Own Health

13.1. When the Therapist Is Ill

13.1.1. Patient Reactions

A therapist's illness brings up fears of separation and abandonment. When the ill therapist cancels sessions, patients may fantasize that the therapist will never return. Or if he does, he will not be able to handle a full practice. And patients may wonder if they will be among those chosen or eliminated in the reduced case load.

Upon the return to practice, immediate transference reactions can appear. Patients often express hostile and aggressive feelings regarding separation and what was experienced as sudden abandonment. Or they are depressed and feel disappointed at the therapist for being weak. And, there are the feelings of guilt at possibly being a burden, or in some way a cause of the illness.

A patient whose family had a history of cancer, for example, fantasized that he was responsible for his therapist's illness (a corneal dysplasia) and feared that the illness would pass on to him. In addition, feelings that he was safe in therapy disappeared when he saw that the therapist could not even protect himself (Kriechman, 1984).

Another patient, whose father had traveled for prolonged periods, adopted a defensive attitude of "conscious indifference" to the separation caused by her therapist's cancellations for his illness (Dewald, 1982). She responded in the same way as she had to her father's absences: verbalizing "realistically appropriate" concerns but repressing and denying emotions related to both relationships.

Ideally, the therapist should be able to observe the patient's reactions to gain a better understanding of the way the patient handles loss and secrecy, and how these issues were dealt with by the patient's parents. As much as possible, the therapist can help patients analyze and integrate the meaning of their reactions to the therapist's illness.

13.1.2. The Therapist's Own Reactions

When an illness seriously threatens life or is in some way chronically debilitating, therapists, like other individuals, utilize the usual defenses of denial and isolation. Often the therapists' and the patients' denials reinforce each other, helping both to defend against facing the issues of the therapists' vulnerability, lack of being special, impotence, and not being able to take care of themselves or their patients (Halpert, 1982).

One of the most extensive discussions of a therapist's illness is that presented by Dewald (1982). Dewald was hospitalized for six weeks for what turned out to be a nearly fatal intracranial infection, which was followed by a one-month convalescence. Upon returning to work he had an oculomotor palsy and had to wear an eye patch (see also Kriechman, 1984, regarding patient reactions to an eye patch). When Dewald first went into the hospital, he had his secretary call patients to tell them that he was ill and would be back at work in a week. The second week he did the same thing. Upon later analysis he felt that this was his own denial operating regarding the seriousness of his condition. In terms of his countertransference, he felt he also wanted to reassure his patients and to protect them. As the illness progressed, the patients were told that he would be away from practice indefinitely and would contact them when he was ready to return to work. As his illness worsened, Dewald felt in retrospect that his sense of responsibility and concern for his patients' welfare lessened, as did his concern regarding his own loss of income and medical expenses. He felt that as his regression deepened, he became increasingly self-centered and preoccupied.

Besides experiencing illness as a threat to the body's integrity, therapists have special concerns related to their profession. First, there is the concern about the ability to continue practicing one's profession: Will I be able to earn a living? Will others still refer patients to me? Will patients stay with me? Will I be able to do my work, to maintain standards, to remain alert, empathetic, neutral, and objective in the face of pain, discomfort, weakness, or other impairments (Halpert, 1982)?

13.1.2.1. Continuing to Work

A therapist may find it helpful in fighting off the disease to continue working and not to give in to the illness. However, when faced with a debilitating disease or the possibility of death, to continue working may impose "an unnecessary and destructive burden on the patient" (Halpert,

1982). For one, the physical and mental changes in the therapist may make it difficult for the patient to raise personal issues that seem trivial in relation to what is happening to the therapist. And as the illness progresses, the therapist may become preoccupied with his or her own difficulties and not be appropriately available to the patient.

Although it may be preferable for the therapy to be terminated before it becomes disturbing, the point may be reached more suddenly than expected, or so gradually that the therapist is not aware of the effect it is having. And the therapist's own physicians may not be totally open about the prognosis, thus supporting denial and nurturing hope.

Therapists have an early model for the stoic approach in the face of serious illness. Freud was chronically ill with oral cancer for the last 17 years of his life. He continued working for most of this time, during which he suffered pain, underwent numerous surgeries, and had a noticeable facial deformity as a result. Halpert (1982) suggests that Freud's famous Wolf Man patient may have strongly reacted to Freud's illness. However, it is interesting that Freud himself did not write about the effects of his illness on therapy, which leads to the assumption that he may have been making extensive use of denial.

13.1.2.2. Returning to Work

Following a serious illness, the questions of when and if to return to work have ethical and psychological implications, in addition to medical ones. There is always the possibility that the therapist will try to return to work prematurely. As recuperation begins to take place and strength begins to return, there may be a need to reestablish self-esteem, to prove oneself competent and intact. However, the residual effects of the illness can interfere with optimal functioning, and one's appearance may be upsetting to patients. The convalescing therapist may have to contend with inarticulateness, memory distortions, inability to concentrate, and pain. Personal issues can invade consciousness, even when one resumes work on a part-time basis, and the self-absorption may interfere with the clinical skill needed.

For those doing psychodynamic or psychoanalytic work, one of the goals of therapy upon returning to work is to explore the full gamut of the patients' responses, affects, and associations to the separation and/or illness. Recently ill therapists may be tempted to avoid this, partly out of their own feelings of vulnerability. However, if the problem is not discussed, the progress of therapy may be impeded, and the patient may begin to act out. Reactions to the illness are not limited to the period immediately following the return to work but may resurface periodically. It may take months or even years to work through the issues that have been stirred up.

13.2. THE DEATH OF A THERAPIST

Shwed (1980) reported that patients' reactions to the unexpected death of their psychiatrist followed expected patterns for grief and mourning. Initially, some were able to vent their deeply felt loss by crying and sharing their fears and anxieties; others developed somatic complaints or reacted with what was described as stoic acceptance or denial. After the initial period of mourning, other feelings began to emerge: anger, feelings of rejection and abandonment. Some of these emotions were directed toward the deceased therapist, others toward the new therapist, who was judged to be less experienced and therefore less competent. Unexpectedly, some families and friends of the patients exhibited intense hostility toward the deceased. In some cases they may have resented the patient's close relationship with the therapist, being envious or feeling left out of the important relationship. Others may have felt displaced or impotent at not being able to help the patient, as the therapist had done. These reactions serve as a warning against assuming that patients can expect to receive emotional support and understanding from those close to them, should their therapist die.

Lord, Ritvo, and Solnit (1978) surveyed 27 patients whose analysts had died in the midst of treatment. Reactions were more pronounced if the therapist died suddenly than if death had followed several months of illness. This suggests that during the period of illness, the patients had had time to work on issues of separation and loss, and thus were more prepared. Severe reactions, such as prolonged mourning, were noted in those who were older, who had been in treatment longer, and who had had a number of early losses, separations, deprivations, and abandonments in their lives.

Rothman, a gynecologist and psychotherapist, kept extensive notes on his patients' reactions and his own countertransference feelings following his diagnosis of lymphoma at age 69 (Kaplan & Rothman, 1986). Rothman first underwent surgery that involved his right kidney. Subsequently he received radiation and chemotherapy, which caused him to miss occasional appointments with patients. About four months following the first surgery, he had a lymph node dissection in his neck, which left him for a time with visible bandages. Two months after the lymph node dissection, his hair fell out as the result of the chemotherapy. Patients' reactions at this time were quite severe. Some exhibited mourning and depression, i.e., staying in bed and missing work. Others experienced intense anxiety over the threat of separation. One woman patient reacted with acute panic and screamed at Dr. Rothman, insisting that he should have cancelled the appointment.

Although, according to Rothman's notes, all his patients were informed of his condition, the patients themselves each remembered the period differently. Following his death, when patients were interviewed by his colleague, Dr. Kaplan, some claimed not to have been told anything; others stated that Dr. Rothman kept reassuring them that all would be well and they clung to this hope. Some of the patients felt that his own optimism encouraged them to deny the reality of the situation. Later, they reacted with anger and sadness that they were not able to begin mourning for him while he was alive. However, it is important to bear in mind that what patients remember is often distorted by their own needs and past history. Later, some of Rothman's patients reported that their eventual mourning of his death had been helpful for them in their later therapy because they were able to work through repressed grief reactions to earlier losses in their lives.

13.3. SELF-DISCLOSURE

There is a wide difference in opinion on the amount of self-disclosure permitted, going from the extreme in some self-encounter groups to almost none in traditional psychoanalysis. Rather than focusing on whether or not to disclose the information, the decision should focus on what revealing or not revealing would mean to individual patients (Flaherty, 1979; Givelber & Simon, 1981). "To tell or not to tell...neither is neutral and either will have important unintended effects" (Gill, cited in Givelber & Simon, 1981).

13.3.1. Factors to Consider in Disclosure

What and how much to share depends upon a host of factors, some of which are specific to the therapist (Flaherty, 1979; Givelber & Simon, 1981). These include (1) the therapist's temperament and personality style, (2) the therapist's background and training, (3) the therapist's previous stance on sharing personal information, and (4) the general degree of comfort or anxiety the therapist may experience with the disclosure.

Patient variables also need to be taken into account (Dewald, 1982; Flaherty, 1979; Givelber & Simon, 1981): the patient's character and pathology, including the degree of reality testing; the patient's interest in learning about the therapist's personal life; the specific information involved; and the amount and kind of factual information the patient has had about the illness.

Also important are the type of therapy, the stage of therapy, and the transference at the time of the proposed disclosure. After returning to work, Dewald (1982), as a psychoanalyst, provided information based on the type of therapy being provided and the stage of analysis. Those seen for supportive or superficial psychotherapy received the most immediate and detailed information and answers to their questions. This was done because the therapeutic strategy was to minimize conscious awareness of transference distortions, fantasies, and responses. Those in the early phase of psychoanalysis received moderate amounts of information. Those in the middle phase received the least factual information and the greatest encouragement to expose and explore transference-inspired distortions and reactions. Those in the termination phase were able to resume analytic work and were able to explore fantasies without information from their analyst.

13.3.2. The Parent–Child Relationship

When the illness is acute and the therapist expects to return to work, giving too much detailed information may interfere with subsequent analysis of the patients' fantasies and affective reactions to the illness. On the other hand, giving essentially no factual information may leave patients with their fears, causing a great deal of upset when sessions are canceled.

Both sharing and not sharing one's experiences, however, may mimic a pattern from the patient's childhood and may be reacted to as such. The patient/child may have felt burdened by the parent who turned to the child for parental help. If the situation is reminiscent of the earlier experiences, old resentments may resurface, with the therapist unexpectedly becoming the focus of anger, hostility, or other extreme emotions.

A delicate balance exists between openness that is helpful and openness that is overwhelming. In comparing disclosure in therapy with a parent–child relationship, Givelber and Simon (1981) feel that under some conditions, a parent's being open with a child can validate the child's perception, encourage communication, and indicate that the parent has confidence in the child's ability to deal with the information and the event. In other circumstances, parental sharing can be seductive or exploitative.

To exclude the patient from discussion does not necessarily protect the patient, particularly if the patient knows or suspects something (Flaherty, 1979; Halpert, 1982; Kaplan & Rothman, 1986). This too may mimic earlier family patterns and prohibitions. The patient may feel confused and insecure, not knowing what is happening, and believing that the subject is a forbidden topic.

13.3.3. Countertransference

Abend (1982) takes issue with the suggestion of sharing personal information with patients. He cautions that countertransference issues may be at the core of most sharing, even though the therapist may claim that knowing is for the good of the patient. Thus, it may be easier for the therapist to share personal information than to deal with patients' fully expressed feelings and fantasies. By trying to be more of a person, a therapist may unconsciously be looking for care, love, and comfort from patients, thereby putting his or her own needs first. Not all patients can or want to handle this closeness. It is important to remember that it is still a therapeutic relationship, and some consistency in the way the sessions are conducted is needed.

Telling can convey hidden countertransference messages. Although most therapists would not directly ask patients to worry about them when they are sick, or ask patients not be angry with them for missing sessions, this may be implicit when sharing the personal information.

On the other hand, the therapists' own resistance to discussing their own illness may stem from several sources. The patients' associations may stir up painful memories, and there may be doubts about the extent of one's own recovery and the ability to function properly. The therapist may be experiencing guilt for the patients' emotional turmoil during the separation, or may be having difficulty tolerating the patients' anger and aggression that surface following the resumption of work.

Also, when interpreting the patients' resistance to discussing the illness, therapists must be careful that they are not trying to fulfill personal needs, i.e., wanting to be missed, reinforcing their own importance to the patient, or using the patient to express their own unresolved anxieties. Ideally, therapists should possess both the capacity and the maturity to assess their own situation accurately, and to place patients' welfare above their own comfort—but this is not always humanly possible.

What and when to tell may really be academic questions. Usually there is not a great deal of control when severe illness or an accident occurs. When a therapist is in the throes of illness and treatment, decisions may be communicated to patients by others, who are in no position to anticipate the meaning this might have for the patients or the patients' emotional reactions. Patients may gain information about the therapist from sources other than the therapist or those designated to speak on the therapist's behalf. For example, sometimes information appears in the local paper, or the patient knows someone who works in the hospital where the ill therapist is being treated. What a patient hears and retains is influenced to a large extent by transference factors. Not knowing exactly what was said to each patient by those acting as intermediaries can complicate the therapy when it resumes.

13.4. PREPARATION FOR ILLNESS AND DEATH

Because of the nature of their work, therapists may be less prone to think of their own illness or death, or other crises that might befall them. Chernin (1976) has written about the therapist's feelings of omnipotence, of being the one who takes care of others, who is in control. This is especially true for psychiatrists, who, as physicians, may feel "magically protected from diseases and disabilities" (Kriechman, 1984). Illness often catches both therapist and patient by surprise.

Some suggest that consulting with a colleague or supervisor can be helpful in trying to handle one's own illness or other personal difficulties.

This can be helpful in facing the seriousness of the illness, and in figuring out the best ways to tell patients, according to their individual needs and readiness (Kaplan & Rothman, 1986). The assumption is, however, that the colleague will be able to be direct with the ill therapist. It is not easy to tell people that they can no longer function as they once did. And colleagues may not even be sure of how to assess the situation or, because of their own defenses and projections, may not be able to face the seriousness of the other's condition.

13.4.1. Planned Termination

Some therapists recommend planned termination of treatment before the therapist becomes incapacitated (Halpert, 1982; Kaplan & Rothman, 1986), particularly if death is expected. This makes it possible for the patients to work through emotions that accompany the loss and mourning, and it facilitates transfer to another therapist while the first therapist is still alive. Planned termination, however, assumes that the therapist is able to come to terms with his or her own impending death. At what point does this take place? With some potentially fatal illnesses, the person has many healthy months or years before succumbing to the disease. It also assumes that patients will want to transfer to another therapist. Some may show resistance, preferring to stay with the ill therapist to the end, and prolonging the eventual separation. If the therapist gives a referral to another therapist before the actual working through of the separation has been achieved, the anger at the abandonment may be transferred onto the next therapist, and further therapeutic work may not be possible, at least for some time.

IV

Psychological Interventions:
Empirical and Theoretical Approaches

14

Psychodynamic and
Supportive Psychotherapy

14.1. THERAPY AND PATIENT MANAGEMENT

Attention to medical patients' emotional states or psychic conflicts has a
beneficial effect on their overall management (Smith, Glass & Miller, 1980;
Thompson & Thompson, 1985). When patients internalize anxiety, for example, this can lead to physiological symptoms, such as high blood pressure and increased pulse or gastrointestinal problems (Rotman *et al.*, 1977).
And interventions that help the patient identify the source of the stress and
deal with the anxiety can have a positive effect on the body.

In this era of economic parsimony, it is important to note that the use of
psychological services has been shown to result in a reduction in the use of
medical facilities, as well as in the number of presenting medical problems
(Follette & Cummings, 1967; Goldberg, Krantz, & Locke, 1970; Rosen &
Wiens, 1979).

Besides the benefit to patients' emotional and physical well-being, a
psychological evaluation can help the physician reevaluate a patient's unexplained behavior and complaints, reducing the need for subsequent medical visits (Rosen & Wiens, 1979). Also, psychological interventions have the
advantage that they are less invasive than drugs and other medical forms of
treatment. And patients are often more willing to reveal their emotional
needs and fears to mental health professionals, who are expected to ask
personal questions, whereas a ''stiff upper lip'' may be shown to the busy
medical staff.

14.2. INDIVIDUAL PSYCHOTHERAPY

In the initial stages of an illness, as well as in the final stages of a
terminal disease, supportive therapy plays an important role. Patients have

fears that they do not wish to share with family or friends, and need a place to cry, to complain, to be understood. Often they feel that others cannot fully appreciate their distress, or cannot abide their continuing need to talk about their difficulties. The therapist lends emotional support and encouragement, as well as education. During these crisis periods, patients feel overwhelmed and need to keep their defenses in check.

During prolonged hospitalization and the subsequent treatment for chronic illness, dynamic psychotherapy can help patients confront the physical and sociocultural changes that occur (Moran, 1985). Following the initial period of shock, patients may need to overcome defenses that are getting in the way of recovery. Often a preexisting personality disorder confounds the adjustment process, and through psychotherapy the patient learns new coping strategies.

Problems stemming from the illness may touch upon unconscious fears, producing emotional reactions and behaviors that the medical staff are unable to handle. In dynamic therapy, patients deal with the deeper issues of self-image, sex, suffering, and death. They also examine issues related to their eventual reentry into the social and vocational world. A transference relationship develops that is useful in helping patients understand their struggles with issues such as dependency, authority, and separation. Through "talking therapy" patients begin to understand the historical basis of their fears and conflicts, and thus regain a sense of control in their lives. The therapist makes appropriate interpretive remarks, helping the patient gain insight into the psychological issues that interact with the realities of the illness, causing increased emotional discomfort.

14.3. DIFFERENTIAL DIAGNOSIS

Mental health professionals may be consulted when patients exhibit signs of delirium or psychotic behavior. The underlying cause may be psychological, organic, or related to other factors, such as medication. The therapist may be asked to help with the differential diagnosis, as well as to treat the manifest psychological symptoms.

Hayes et al. (1986) describe how the disease itself and the prescribed medication, can produce symptoms that appear on the surface to be psychologically based. This was exemplified by the anxiety, depression, and tremulousness in patients with advanced chronic bronchitis and emphysema, and by the confusion, disorientation, and paranoid ideation in patients with systemic lupus erythematosus.

Following surgery, particularly heart surgery, some patients undergo what has been called "postoperative psychosis." Possible precipitating factors are advanced age, preoperative anxiety and personality factors, the extent of the surgery, time under anesthesia, the kind and amount of medication, alcohol withdrawal, sleep deprivation, and sensory deprivation. An unexplained finding is that those demonstrating personality traits of dominance, aggressiveness, and self-assurance have shown a greater tendency toward postoperative delirium (Rogers & Reich, 1986).

Delirium is a broad term used for any syndrome of disturbed sensation, perception, memory, thought, or judgment resulting from altered cerebral functioning (Heller & Kornfeld, 1975). Physical causes of delirium include bleeding resulting in cerebral anemia, circulatory impairment, metabolic derangement from fluid and electrolyte imbalance, fever, hypoglycemia, liver failure, kidney failure, and metastases, particularly in the case of lung and breast cancer, and acquired immune deficiency syndrome (AIDS).

Patients who have been infected with the AIDS virus (HIV positive), for example, may present with mental status changes due to central nervous system (CNS) involvement. On the other hand, these changes may be psychological reactions to having contracted the disease (Rundell, Wise, & Ursano, 1986). The presenting symptoms are similar. In some cases, paranoia or suspiciousness, delirium, or dementia may be the first indications of CNS problems. A differential diagnosis, making use of psychoneurological tests, can have serious prognostic implications at this point, since CNS involvement often portends the final stages of AIDS (Levy, Pons, & Rosenblum, 1984).

Organic involvement may show up in the form of poor concentration and decreased attention span, difficulty with spelling, a lack of abstract reasoning, impairment in concept formation, and diminished psychomotor speed. In some cases, there may be preexisting emotional problems or an underlying personality disorder that can be detected through the use of structured interviews, objective tests (e.g., the MMPI) and projective devices (e.g., the Rorschach).

14.4. Psychotherapy Interventions: The Research

That psychotherapy can have some effect with some patients has been demonstrated, but the results of studies have been inconsistent (Conte & Karasu, 1981; Kellner, 1975). Differences in outcomes depend upon a host of factors, including the type of intervention, the patient population of interest, and the definition of "successful treatment." Most published research with the physically ill has involved cognitive-behavioral approaches. However, supportive and dynamic interventions are quite common. Some examples from the literature are discussed in the following sections.

14.4.1. Peptic Ulcer Disease

A study of psychotherapy with peptic ulcer disease (PUD) patients has revealed the long-range effects of psychotherapy, and also cautions that these effects may not be immediately obvious (Sjodin, Svedlund, Ottoson, & Dotevall, 1986). Those who underwent individual psychotherapy (10 one-hour sessions over three months), along with their medical treatment, were compared with those who did not have the benefit of therapy (control group). During the course of the treatment, both groups showed improvement, physically and mentally. Had the study ended here, no significant differences would have been found. However, the initial improvement experienced by the control group did not last, and was followed by deterioration once the medical treatment was finished. For those undergoing psychotherapy, the abdominal pain and other somatic symptoms stabilized or got better throughout the 15-month follow-up period. These patients also reported greater self-confidence and an improved ability to cope with life in general. The authors explain the more favorable outcome for the psychotherapy group as their having found more effective ways of coping with stress and emotional problems, as well as having a better understanding and sense of control over their abdominal disorder.

The psychotherapy intervention was dynamically oriented and supportive. The traditional psychodynamic approach was modified for those patients who had difficulty expressing emotions verbally. Therapeutic goals varied from pointing out connections between symptoms and stressors, to dealing with specific dynamic conflicts. Other psychotherapeutic approaches to dealing with catastrophes in life, such as illness, have been described by Druss (1986) and Kanas, Kaltreider, and Horowitz (1977).

14.4.2. Cardiac Disease

Gruen (1975) reported that daily supportive individual psychotherapy with post-myocardial-infarction (heart attack) inpatients resulted in less depression, less anxiety, and fewer physical symptoms. A four-month follow-up revealed that these patients had spent fewer days in intensive care and in the hospital and had suffered fewer episodes of congestive heart failure and supraventricular arrhythmias. They also had a more positive social orientation and had returned more quickly to a normal level of activity.

In a later study, over 800 victims of heart attacks were randomly assigned to two groups—i.e., the treatment group, which received psychological counseling to reduce Type A characteristics, and the control group, which did not (Friedman et al., 1984). Over a three-year period, those receiving counseling had a significantly reduced rate of recurrence of nonfatal heart attacks. The psychological interventions used included supportive therapy along with behavior/cognitive techniques.

14.4.3. Cancer

A study of cancer patients (lung, breast, melanoma) who had received short-term psychotherapy (on the average, 11 20-minute sessions in the hospital) showed improvement related to psychological interventions (Gordon et al., 1980). The counseling focused on the patient's emotional reactions toward having cancer, and included an educational component. Although the results were mixed, patients who participated in psychotherapy evidenced a more rapid decline in anxiety, hostility, and depression, as compared with controls. They also reported a more realistic outlook on life and had a more active usage of their time after discharge, and a greater proportion of them returned to their previous level of work. The particular site of the cancer was found to be an important variable associated with different body image concerns, different reactions to medical treatment, and different degrees of need for psychological services. Those with lung cancer, for example, required more visits, on the average, from the psychological counselor, and those with melanoma the least.

The stage of the illness is a crucial factor in determining the effect of psychotherapy. Cassileth, Lusk, Miller, Brown, and Miller (1985) did not find psychotherapy to have any significant effect on the length of survival or time to relapse for patients in the late stages of cancer. However, once a certain point has been reached, even medical treatments may have little or no effect on reversing the disease process. But these factors are not the only criteria for evaluating the benefits of psychotherapy. The emotional support from the relationship with a caring therapist may be of considerable importance in helping terminal patients face death and deal with the experience of abandonment felt by many during the final stages.

14.4.4. Preoperative Preparation

Psychological preparation is needed for patients facing surgery or medical treatment that is expected to result in severe side effects, or a functional loss or deficit. Such preparation is needed with surgeries such as laryngectomy, colostomy, orchiectomy, and mastectomy, and with treatments such as chemotherapy, radiation, and dialysis. An understanding of which effects will be permanent and which temporary is crucial. Concerns about possible sexual dysfunction need to be discussed as openly as possible.

In a review of the literature, Rogers and Reich (1986) reported that brief preoperative interviewing with a psychiatrist or psychologist can reduce the incidence of postoperative psychosis. In some cases where psychoticlike behavior has occurred, patients who had the benefit of psychological intervention, including being informed about the possibility of unusual perceptual disturbances, reported feeling more comfortable and more in control when confronted with these experiences than did patients who had no received the counseling.

A review of 34 controlled studies revealed that surgical or medical patients who are provided with information or emotional support at the time of a medical crisis have a better outcome (e.g., shorter length of stay in the hospital) than do patients who receive traditional routine medical care (Mumford, Schlesinger, & Glass, 1982). Often a positive effect is achieved in only one or two visits, a highly cost-effective intervention.

In an early study by Egbert, Battit, Welch, and Bartlett (1964), patients were visited the night before surgery by the anesthesiologist, who reassured them and provided information. This simple intervention reduced significantly the amount of pain and the need for postoperative morphine, as well as the number of days in the hospital. In another study (Dumas & Leonard, 1963), postoperative vomiting was reduced for those patients who had been visited one hour before surgery by a nurse who remained with them until the moment of anesthesia.

Cooperation during cardiac catheterization was improved by preparing patients with both specific information and emotional support—taking only two sessions, one the day before the procedure and one on the day of surgery (Rogers & Reich, 1986). The largest effect was in the reduction of psychotropic medication.

Research suggests that giving information about what the patient might experience results in a more calming effect than simply providing technical information. However, not all patients react the same way to preoperative preparations (e.g., the giving of information regarding the procedure). Some negative effects have been reported in patients designated as "deniers" or "avoiders," who generally have a slower recovery rate (see Chapter 12).

In general, however, a person's perception of how well he or she is doing affects improvement (Garrity, 1973a, 1973b, 1975). But the perception of health status does not always coincide with the actual condition. Psychological interventions designed to improve patients' understanding of their illness can be effective in changing their perceptions of what is to come and how well they are doing, thus affecting morale and influencing subsequent behavior in a positive direction.

15

Cognitive–Behavior Therapy

Cognitive–behavior techniques have been applied to alleviate physical pain, anxiety, and maladaptive adjustments related to physical illness. Although distinctions are made between the behavioral and cognitive approaches, the techniques overlap and are often used in conjunction with one another.

Behavioral therapy involves behavioral modification, such as positive and negative reinforcement through biofeedback (Beck, Rush, Shaw, & Emery, 1979; Burish & Bradley, 1983; Turk & Rudy, 1986; Wolpe, 1974). In the case of physical illness, the unwanted symptoms (e.g., anxiety responses, pain) are thought of as learned habits, which can be retrained or progressively diminished by repeated exposure to a competing response (Wolpe, 1980).

Cognitive therapy focuses on identifying and correcting distorted cognitions, controlling unwanted thoughts and behaviors, and developing alternative behaviors or strategies for coping with illness. Patients are taught to monitor covert and overt events that precede, accompany, and follow stressful situations. They learn to employ selected coping skills to combat anxiety-arousing rumination, to apply rational problem-solving techniques to practical problems (e.g., self-assertion), to reappraise anxiety-provoking events, to make use of calm self-talk, and to control unwanted thoughts and feelings through selective attention (Langer, Janis, & Wolfer, 1975).

In preoperative preparation, cognitive techniques were found to be more efficacious than providing information alone. With just a 20-minute session, a psychologist was able to reduce the percentage of patients requesting sedatives, as well as reducing the total number of analgesics used. The special coping techniques that were taught included cognitive reappraisal of anxiety-provoking events, calm self-talk, and cognitive control through selective attention (Langer *et al.*, 1975).

Both behavior and cognitive psychologists make use of relaxation techniques (Davis, Eshelman, & McKay, 1980). These include exercises, such as progressive muscle relaxation, where the patient is instructed to concentrate on specified muscle groups, tightening them, then relaxing them, gradually moving from one part of the body to another (e.g., starting with the feet and working up to the head). The intent is to produce a subjective state of calm, something that can also be achieved through hypnosis, suggestion, and transcendental meditation (Wallace, 1970). Progressive muscle relaxation can be used by tense patients who are having difficulty sleeping because of obsessive thoughts about their illness.

With imagery, another form of relaxation, the patient is asked to focus on the sensory details of a pleasant scene. Simonton, Matthews-Simonton, and Creighton (1978) and Simonton, Matthews-Simonton, and Sparks (1980) have developed methods of imagery for treating cancer. For example, patients learn to focus on thoughts of cure (e.g., chasing the disease from the body by means of a large imaginary shiny ball). Some respond positively to this technique, at least on an emotional level, feeling that they are doing something about the illness, that they are finally taking charge in a time when everything is out of their control. Supporters who use these methods claim to have had actual cures; however, replication through controlled studies is needed.

One interesting study (Roth & Holmes, 1987) found that aerobic exercises were more effective than relaxation training, not only in improving cardiovascular fitness but in reducing the severity and duration of depression following stressful life events. No differences were found, however, between the two methods on self-report of physical health.

15.1. THE TERMINALLY ILL

Cognitive training and imagery have been used with dying patients in order to disrupt disturbing thoughts, feelings, and behaviors (Sobel, 1981). Patients are encouraged to focus on images, faces, events, landscapes, or memories that elicit warm and happy feelings (Preston, 1973). There is no research to demonstrate its effectiveness, and some professionals have voiced reservations, implying that the approach is disrespectful, and cautioning that the techniques may strengthen the defense of denial at a time when the patient could benefit more from working through issues related to death (S.M. Levy, 1983).

15.2. PSYCHOSOMATIC ILLNESS

Wolpe (1980) describes the use of behavioral techniques with psychosomatic illnesses, such as asthma, peptic ulcer, irritable colon, migraine headaches, hypertension, and neurodermatitis. These illnesses are commonly thought to have emotional underpinnings, or to be triggered by external stimuli.

Bennett and Wilkinson (1985), for example, found that stress management training based on progressive muscle relaxation and self-instructional training was more effective than medication alone in treating irritable bowel syndrome (IBS). Subjects were seen individually for one hour at weekly intervals, with homework assignments between sessions. Those in the medical treatment group were seen only once a month. Psychological intervention was shown to reduce both anxiety and IBS symptoms over a period of eight weeks. It is not clear from the study, however, if it was the supportive environment of the once-a-week meeting or the particular type of psychotherapy technique used. Also, results were based on only 12 subjects, so replication of the study is needed before generalizations can be made with confidence.

Others have looked at psychological interventions to decrease the incidence of heart attack. In one report, a meta-analysis of 18 studies lends support to the contention that cognitive–behavioral interventions can be used to modify Type A behavior and thus reduce the possibility of heart attack (Nunes, Frank, & Kornfeld, 1987). Some of the interventions used by Nunes *et al.* are illustrative of the different methods:

1. *Education*—providing information about chronic heart disease and coronary-prone behavior (Type A).
2. *Relaxation exercises*—training in imagery and progressive muscle relaxation, as well as yoga.
3. *Cognitive restructuring*—modifying exaggerated emotional reactions and Type A thoughts, e.g., changing "I have to get there faster" to "I'm going fast enough."
4. *Imagining*—thinking about arousing situations and confrontations from everyday life, and then imagining appropriate coping skills, such as relaxation or cognitive restructuring.
5. *Behavior modification*—rehearsing desired behavior through role playing, or practicing behavioral prescriptions between sessions, and establishing new values and goals.
6. *Psychodynamic interventions*—encouraging subjects to ventilate their painful feelings and experiences in a supportive environment, and making dynamic interpretations of their unconscious motives and conflicts underlying the Type A behavior.

The results of the Nunes *et al.* study revealed that combinations of these cognitive–behavioral techniques, along with the psychodynamic interventions, are more effective than a given technique used alone (also in Holroyd, 1986).

15.3. IMPROVING COMPLIANCE

Behavioral management techniques have been found to be effective in combatting noncompliance with diabetic and asthmatic patients. For example, assertiveness training has helped diabetic patients in the management of their disease by enabling them to confront medical staff with their questions and needs (Rabin *et al.*, 1986). Also of importance to the issue of compliance is the ability through training for patients to view criticism as constructive, rather than having it adversely affect their self-esteem (Stoudemire, 1985). Although the behavioral management of the physical symptoms of asthma has not been encouraging, these techniques have been used to reduce the amount of maladaptive behavior, such as noncompliance, malingering, and deliberate provocation of attacks (Stoudemire, 1985).

15.4. CONDITIONED RESPONSES TO CHEMOTHERAPY

Some patients develop a conditioned negative response (à la Pavlov) to chemotherapy. Sights, sounds, smells, tastes, even thoughts associated with the administration of the drugs can elicit nausea and vomiting prior to treatment (Morrow, 1982; Nesse, Carli, Curtis, & Kleinman, 1980). A majority of patients undergoing chemotherapy will probably experience some anticipatory reactions (Olafsdottir, Sjoden, & Westling, 1986).

Patients who develop anticipatory nausea and vomiting (CNV), when compared with those who do not, have been characterized as having had more severe postinjection nausea and vomiting, a greater number of chemotherapy sessions, more time-consuming chemotherapy infusions, and stronger taste sensations. They have also been treated with agents with high emetic potential, and have experienced more anxiety during treatment (Andrykowski & Redd, 1985, 1987; Olafsdottir *et al.*, 1986).

Since CNV is highly resistant to antiemetic drugs, behavioral interventions have been used in attempting to reduce or eliminate these negative conditioned responses (Burish & Carey, 1984). Although many patients benefit from the techniques (e.g., progressive muscle relaxation, systemic desensitization, hypnosis, electromyographic EEG biofeedback, and skin temperature biofeedback), others do not (Burish, Shartner, & Lyles, 1981; Lyles, Burish, Krozely, & Oldham, 1982; Morrow & Morrell, 1982; Redd, Andersen, & Minagawa, 1982). Carey and Burish (1985), in studying ways to decrease negative anticipatory responses, found that those with low levels of anxiety benefited most from the behavioral training. These patients exhibited a significantly greater reduction in anxiety, depression, and diastolic blood pressure. These surprising results suggest that highly anxious patients are the least likely to benefit from behavioral treatments aimed at reducing conditioned negative responses to chemotherapy. The researchers speculate that patients with moderate or high anxiety may have more difficulty concentrating and thus are unable to learn the behavioral techniques effectively.

Most efforts have been directed toward reducing the frequency and severity of symptoms. However, Burish, Carey, Krozely, and Greco (1987) found that training in relaxation techniques and guided imagery, prior to the beginning of chemotherapy and during the first three sessions, was able to prevent, or at least retard, CNV responses. These behavioral techniques were also effective in reducing the conditioned side effects that occur during the 72 hours that immediately follow chemotherapy. The study followed the patients and the controls through only five chemotherapy sessions; however, the researchers feel that since the techniques can be self-administered, they would have some effect on conditioned symptoms that might develop later on. These results suggest that patients would probably benefit from training in relaxation techniques and imagery prior to the development of CNV, rather than waiting for side effects to occur.

15.5. NEUROLOGICAL AND NEUROMUSCULAR DISORDERS

Biofeedback and other behavior techniques have been attempted in the treatment of various neurological and neuromuscular disorders. A review of the literature on these interventions, however, reveals a dearth of rigorous empirical studies and only equivocal results (Parker & Baer, 1986). For example, self-control of seizures has revealed anecdotal success, but the results of research are mixed. Biofeedback, self-hypnosis, and imagery have been used with some, albeit limited, success in the control of phantom limb pain following amputation. Studies of behavioral management of cerebral trauma patients have been plagued by poor research design and few or no follow-up data. What is observed in the laboratory during training does not necessarily translate into practical or long-term effectiveness.

15.6. BEHAVIORAL MANAGEMENT RESEARCH: THE DEBATE

Although there is a great deal of research published in the area of behavioral management of the physically ill, most has suffered from serious methodological problems, and the overall results are not conclusive. Proponents of cognitive–behavioral techniques frequently claim success; however, there needs to be more replication of studies, more controlled research with larger samples, and more long-term follow-up studies (Burish & Bradley, 1983). Roberts (1985, 1986) has questioned the effectiveness of biofeedback in particular, suggesting that it does not replace the special relationship between therapist and patient. His criticisms, needless to say, have resulted in much debate (Green & Shellenberger, 1986; McGovern, 1986; Norris, 1986; Smith, 1986; White & Tursky, 1986).

In support of Roberts, though possibly unintentionally, is the large volume covering studies of behavioral management of chronic diseases, edited by Burish and Bradley (1983). Although each chapter is filled with citations of research on behavior–cognitive interventions, the chapter summaries inevitably consider much of the research anecdotal or suffering from serious methodological weaknesses. The limitations restrict the extent to which one can make generalizations about the effectiveness of the techniques. Despite the severe limitations, some research has demonstrated success and suggests areas for further productive investigation.

16

Group Therapy

Group therapy has been used as an adjunct to medical treatment with a variety of physical illnesses and disabilities (see Table 2). The primary aim of this approach is to help the physically ill patient reduce feelings of anxiety and isolation, and increase their self-acceptance and self-esteem (Singler, 1977). This goal is accomplished by sharing feelings and ideas, and by exchanging information about their medical conditions and treatment. For example, stroke patients who participated in short-term therapy were primarily concerned with physical function, including mobility, driving, and doing housework. Psychological issues also surfaced, related to their care at the rehabilitation center, their expectations about their progress, and their reactions to the stroke (Bucher, Smith, & Gillespie, 1984).

Patients often look to group therapy as a source of social support. Having a good social network has been shown to play an important role in reducing psychological distress and the likelihood of developing a serious illness, as well as enhancing the prospects of recovery for those who are ill (Taylor, Falke, Shoptaw, & Lichtman, 1986). This may explain the finding that those who participated in group therapy following a heart attack have lower mortality and morbidity rates (e.g., Ibrahim *et al.*, 1974; Rahe, O'Neil, Hagan, & Arthur, 1975; Rahe, Ward, & Hayes, 1979).

Essentially, there are four basic types of groups: (1) psychodynamic, (2) cognitive–behavioral, (3) psychoeducational, and (4) self-help groups that do not involve professional leaders. Although a given group may draw upon different approaches, emotional support is perceived as being more helpful than simply receiving information about the illness. And there is some suggestion in the literature that information and advice may not be experienced as helpful, unless coming from medical caregivers (Abrams, 1966; Dunkel-Schetter, 1984).

Many patients join support groups to vent their frustrations with their medical care (Taylor *et al.*, 1986). Cognitive–behavioral groups have had some success in this area by increasing self-confidence, assertiveness, and

Table 2. Group Therapy: Selected References

Illness	References
Cancer, in general	Ferlic, Goldman, & Kennedy, 1979; Heinrich & Schag, 1985b; Spiegel, Bloom, & Yalom, 1981; Taylor, Falke, Shoptaw, & Lichtman, 1986
Breast cancer	Baider, Amikam, & Kaplan De-Nour, 1984; Vachon, Lyall, Rogers, Cochrane, & Freeman, 1981–1982
Head and neck cancer	Harris, Vogtsberger, & Mattox, 1985
Diabetes	Aveline, McCulloch, & Tattersall, 1985; Oehler-Giarratana & Fitzgerald, 1980; Rabin, Amir, Nardi, & Ovadia, 1986; Tattersall, McCulloch, & Aveline, 1985
Genital herpes	Drob & Bernard, 1986
Heart attack	Ibrahim et al, 1974; Rahe, O'Neil, Hagan, & Arthur, 1975; Rahe, Ward, & Hayes, 1979
Hemophilia	Caldwell & Leveque, 1974
Lung disease	Pattison, Rhodes, & Dudley, 1971
Myasthenia gravis	Schwartz & Cahill, 1971
Pain	Moore & Chaney, 1985
Polio	Bozarth, 1987; Laurie & Raymond, 1985
Rheumatoid arthritis	Udelman & Udelman, 1978
Stroke	Bucher, Smith, & Gillespie, 1984; Oradei & Waite, 1974; Piscor & Paleos, 1968; Singler, 1975, 1977, 1981; Spiegel, 1979
Terminal illness	Spiegel, Bloom, & Yalom, 1981; Yalom & Grooves, 1977

compliance. In one study (Rabin et al., 1986), diabetic patients were given assertiveness training to enable them to make demands of the medical staff, such as initiating and insisting upon continuous contact with one primary physician (something found to be predictive of compliance). They were also taught thought-substitution as a way to increase self-confidence by reducing negative thoughts and replacing them with positive ones. An example of negative thought would be: "I'm no good. I can't stick to my diet." The substituted positive thought, when the doctor responds gruffly, could be: "He's just trying to help me; I shouldn't take this personally." The authors report that after 12 training sessions, patients were able to change their thinking about their illness and to deal directly with staff and family.

In a psychodynamic group composed of persons who are blind and diabetic, Oehler-Giarratana and Fitzgerald (1980) reported that direct discussion of blindness and social complications facilitated the ability to grieve over past losses. The discussion also aided patients in dealing with the possibility of loss of function in the future, including the ultimate loss of life itself. Denial was present at first; however, as the participants became more comfortable, they expressed relief at being able to talk about concerns that they had not been able to share with their families. Over time, therapy was characterized by more honesty, awareness, and involvement.

16.1. GROUP CHARACTERISTICS

Although the literature suggests that social support from group therapy can be beneficial, it needs to be kept in mind that most groups are made up of self-selected populations (Taylor *et al.*, 1986). Group therapy is not for everyone. Some patients have found their emotional difficulties intensified by the group sessions. In one study (Baider, Amikam, & Kaplan De-Nour,- 1984), 23% of those contacted refused to participate in a group, giving responses such as "I don't want any more contact with the hospital." "It would depress me, being with all those sick people." "I prefer not to dwell on my illness." Of those who did participate, only half reported a positive benefit.

A study of breast cancer patients suggests that group support may be most helpful for patients with high levels of distress (Vachon, Lyall, Rogers, Cochrane, & Freeman, 1981–1982). On the other hand, a study of adolescents with physical disabilities found that those who terminated group therapy prematurely were more likely to be those whose condition occurred later in life, or whose condition was worsening (Weinman, 1987).

Sex differences have been noted, as well. In the group for stroke patients, Bucher *et al.* (1984) found that the women showed greater anxiety and depression than the men. On weekend leave they would become depressed because they were unable to perform their previous household duties, forcing them to face the reality of their situation. The men, on the other hand, were not ready to return to their jobs and thus had not yet faced the loss of role status. Women also expressed relief at being able to share with others the hostile and guilty feelings they had toward their families. In contrast, the men in the group made use of denial in the form of inappropriate joking and laughing. In general, women tend to prefer groups where there is a sharing of feelings, whereas men prefer psychoeducational groups, particularly when accompanied by their spouses. And, as with mental health services in general, white, upper-middle-class women are the main participants in group therapy.

16.2. GROUP STRUCTURE

Although there is a lack of consensus regarding criteria for group membership, most professionals working with groups favor homogeneity (Chubon, 1982). For example, in a mixed group Singler (1985) found that head-injured patients did not understand, nor could they accept, the stroke patients' fear of a future stroke, and their joint presence in the group tended to inhibit the development of group cohesiveness. Taking an opposite view are those who feel that patients with dissimilar illnesses or disabilities can form viable groups because they often share common problems around issues such as self-esteem, physical appearance, sexuality, and social and family relationships (Dell Orto & Laskey, 1979; Heller, 1970; Marshak, 1982).

Whether or not the groups should be open or closed (i.e., members allowed to join at any time or only in the beginning when the group forms) is an issue that needs further study. Also, the approximate number of sessions required for achieving maximum benefit needs to be clarified. When one is working with the physically ill patient, the scheduling of the group sessions becomes important since patients are more susceptible to fatigue as the day progresses. Thus, groups are more likely to be successful if held earlier in the day (Bucher et al., 1984).

How structured the group sessions themselves should be is another question, and the literature gives contradictory answers. Singler (1981) suggests a directive approach as most useful, whereas, Chubon (1982) favors a nonstructured approach for focusing on immediate needs and allowing members to ventilate anger and frustration and to receive support.

16.3. WHEN A GROUP MEMBER DIES

For patients with advanced or terminal illness, the sharing of anxieties about death and dying seems to lessen fears and improve the overall morale of the group (Spiegel, Bloom, & Yalom, 1981; Yalom & Grooves, 1977). However, there is little in the literature about how to approach the subject of death in groups comprising patients who are in the early stages of illness. Hyland et al., (1984) faced this problem with a group of breast cancer patients. When one of the participants' health began to deteriorate, she became more and more depressed and began to withdraw. The group mirrored her alienation by avoiding any discussion of her symptoms or prognosis. Eventually she did die. Process notes revealed that, although members occasionally brought up the issue of death, it was not discussed. The counselors later revealed that they themselves were hesitant to discuss the subject of death for fear of upsetting the patients. Psychologically they experienced the member's death as a failure, since the aim of the group had been to improve the quality of the patients' lives. These findings should caution group leaders to be aware of their own inhibitions, and to recognize that protectiveness may actually be a defense, a form of resistance.

16.4. THE GROUP LEADER

Whether or not the group leader needs to be someone with the illness is a question that has not been answered by research. Traditionally, groups dealing with alcoholics and drug abusers have used peers as leaders, assuming that this is necessary for insight and rapport. Groups for those with AIDS and breast cancer have frequently followed this prescription. Perhaps for lack of sufficient number, leaders of most other groups for the physically ill patient usually have not had the same medical condition as the group members.

One could argue that those who have had the illness would have a better understanding of what the patients are going through. On the other hand, preoccupation with one's own experience may narrow a leader's focus and make it difficult to maintain an appropriate distance. (See Chapter 5 for further discussion of these countertransference issues.) Group leaders need training and supervision to work through unresolved issues they may have about illness, so they can effectively deal with countertransference as it arises. Whether the leaders also have had the specific illness is probably of secondary importance to their other qualifications.

Those interested in joining or starting a group for the physically ill should check with local organizations and foundations concerned with the specific condition, medical centers and hospitals, or the National Self-Help Clearing House (c/o Graduate School and University Center of the City University of New York, 33 West 42nd Street, Room 1227, New York, New York 10036).

17

Family Therapy

The literature on family therapy with the physically ill includes family systems approaches as well as family and couples counseling (Burr, Good, & Del Veccio-Good, 1978; Huberty, 1974; Moore & Chaney, 1985; Thompson & Thompson, 1985). Some of the work has focused on families trying to cope with the illness of a child (e.g., Binger *et al.*, 1969; Grant, 1978; Minuchin *et al.*, 1975; Power & Del Orto, 1980; Turk, 1964). And others have focused on vocational issues, such as helping those with chronic conditions maintain job stability (e.g., epilepsy, Earl, 1986). There is a dearth of empirical data, however, on the effectiveness of family therapy with the physically ill, although clinical experience and anecdotal accounts in the literature suggest that including the family in counseling and information sessions can be beneficial to both the patient and the family members.

17.1. INTERVENTIONS

Family therapy interventions are designed to increase the family's overall ability to communicate and express feelings, to recognize the realities of the disease, to reduce excessive chaos in daily family functioning, and to learn how to deal with other people's reactions. Some behavioral tactics learned in family therapy may involve helping the family members become more assertive—for example, seeking out doctors, asking questions, finding information about the disease, mobilizing other family members, and learning about community resources.

Certain diseases, such as AIDS, have made it necessary to bring family therapy into the patient's life outside the therapy room. Therapists and counselors find it necessary to go to the patient at home or in the hospital, and to become involved more intensively with the family than in the traditional family therapy models (Walker, 1987).

Family members may need to be reassured about the importance of their role, and to have more realistic expectations about what is expected of them. Sometimes they need to be encouraged to take time away from patient care to enjoy themselves or to relax. This is necessary so they can conserve their own energy and health, as well as their emotional stability and perspective. They may fear that the patient will not understand their need to be alone or away. And indeed the patient may not. These are the kinds of issues where family therapy can intervene to help family members appreciate the needs and motivations of others.

In one study, Heinrich and Schag (1985b) made use of the group approach in dealing with couples. They reported that spouses of cancer patients found group sessions particularly supportive and educational. The group process seemed to have a positive impact on the attitudes of the patients and their spouses toward the medical team and the treatment, and participants reported that they were better able to handle stressful situations as a result of techniques learned in the group. Relaxation techniques were seen as particularly helpful in dealing with stress related to illness, and patients were continuing to apply what they learned in the group at the two-month follow-up. The psychosocial adjustment to their illness improved over time for both the group participants and the controls. That both improved may have been related to an attention factor, since the controls also knew they were in a research project and also had extensive contact with the research team. They did not, however, have the benefit of the behavioral–cognitive group experience.

Minuchin was one of the first to apply the techniques of family therapy to the treatment of psychosomatic disorders, particularly in children (Minuchin, 1974; Minuchin et al., 1975; Minuchin, Rosman, & Baker, 1978). He identified two necessary conditions for the development and maintenance of symptoms: a specific family organizational pattern, and a physiological vulnerability in the child. The child's involvement in parental conflicts further reinforces the symptoms. Minuchin and his colleagues describe four family characteristics that contribute to the development of symptoms: enmeshment (i.e., lack of boundaries), rigidity (vs. adaptability), overprotectiveness, and lack of conflict resolution. Although Minuchin's approach to family theory, research, and intervention needs further validation (Kog, Vertommen, & Vandereycken, 1987), it serves as a basis for family interventions where medical illness is of concern.

17.2. Family Reactions to Illness

Although there has been speculation that particular family systems can cause illness, this has not been demonstrated. Rather, it appears that illness elicits responses that have been characteristic of the family's handling of problems and emotions (Stoudemire, 1985).

Families, like individuals, go through a series of stages in response to the illness of a family member (Shapiro, 1986; Ziegler, 1987). Following the initial diagnosis, members react with shock, disbelief, anxiety, denial, or helplessness. Later, feelings of guilt, self-blame, grief, anticipatory mourning, or chronic sorrow come to the fore.

During the initial stages of the disease, many questions emerge about the patient's prognosis and quality of life. Families frequently fear that an illness will be fatal, even when told that the prognosis is good. For example, a physician's recommending radiation may be interpreted as meaning that the patient's condition is hopeless (Rotman *et al.*, 1977). Some may fear that the patient will become radioactive or contaminated. They may not understand that certain symptoms are side effects of treatment (e.g., diarrhea, difficulty swallowing, or anorexia) and interpret them instead as indications that the disease is progressing.

Anger can surface at the patient for being sick, for becoming a burden, for deserting the family, or at the medical staff for discovering the problem and not being able to cure it. Anger may also be expressed at other family members, and frequently at God for letting this happen. Family members feel guilty about their anger, and about thinking about their own needs when someone else is so terribly sick. Some feel responsible for the illness, fearing they may have transmitted it to the patient, genetically or through a virus, or that they demanded too much, or did not take proper care of the patient. They blame themselves for not recognizing the disease earlier, or not forcing the patient to go for an examination sooner.

It has been said that the patient often recovers emotionally long before the spouse (Soloff, 1977–1978). Wives of heart attack patients suffer for long periods from anxiety, depression, anorexia, and insomnia (Mayou, Foster, & Williamson, 1978). Many, even a year after the attack, repress their own needs and feelings for fear of upsetting their spouse (Links & Kaplan, 1980). Some develop "copy-cat" psychosomatic complaints, such as headaches, stomach pains, faintness, and chest tightness—symptoms not unlike those of their husbands (Skeleton & Dominian, 1973; Stern & Pascale, 1979).

Men are susceptible to the stresses of their wives' illnesses as well. In one study, during the period immediately following the wife's mastectomy, 40% of the husbands developed sleep disorders, including nightmares, and some had difficulty concentrating at work (Jamison, Wellisch, & Pasnau, 1978; Wellisch, Jamison, & Pasnau, 1978). Although most women and their spouses seemed to adjust satisfactorily to the mastectomy, marriages that were unstable prior to the operation tended to deteriorate more so afterward.

Cronkite and Moos (1984) found that the family could be both a source of support and a source of stress, depending upon the spouses' traditional ways of coping. Avoidance coping was seen as "taking it out on others," trying to reduce tension by eating more or smoking more, keeping feelings to oneself, and preparing for the worst. Approach coping was defined as taking positive action, trying to find out more about the situation, trying to step back and be more objective, trying to see the positive side of the situation. The interaction of mood, coping style, and physical illness is illustrated by the following finding:

When both partners were above average on avoidance coping, the husband would become particularly depressed about his wife's physical symptoms. If either one, or both, of the partners relied less on avoidance coping, the husband's depression lessened. Thus, if denial and avoidance are used when the wife is ill, the repressed tensions that result have a considerable negative impact on the husband's mood. This study also found that women responded more to environmental events, be they positive or negative, than did the men. Stressful life events, for example, affected the wives' physical symptoms and depression more adversely than their husbands'. And women, who reported more family support, relied less on avoidance coping and showed less depressed mood and physical symptoms, while similar effects were not observed for their husbands.

17.2.1. Secondary Gain

If the patient and the family are firmly enmeshed with each other around the illness, any attempt to alter this by making the patient "better" or by fostering responsibility for their own care may be undermined. Patients may use the illness to control or dominate, or family members may blame the patient and the illness for any familial problems.

Some patients feel that they are loved out of duty, because they are sick rather than for any positive reason. Their acting-out, rage, and depression are reactions to the perceived lack of caring, or guilt for being a drain on financial and emotional resources (Boehnert & Popkin, 1986). If their dependency needs are not being met in other ways, however, the illness becomes a legitimate means for getting care (Thompson & Thompson, 1985).

17.3. ILLNESS AND DEATH IN A PATIENT'S FAMILY

One day a therapy patient may announce that a family member or close friend has just developed a serious illness or had a disabling accident. As in any traditional psychotherapy, do not assume stereotypical reactions on the patient's part, since there may be ambivalent feelings toward the person who is physically ill. For example, the patient may have been contemplating a divorce, and now finds himself in the role of caretaker. There may also be an increase in the therapy patient's own physical complaints arising from identification with the other, fear of contracting the illness, or guilt (Barsky & Klerman, 1983; Mechanic, 1972).

Brain injury is an example of a chronic condition that creates complicated adjustment problems for those involved with the injured person. The healthy spouse—a wife, for example—may be the person in psychotherapy. She now has to learn to deal with the significant cognitive and behavioral changes that are occurring in her partner, changes that can range from decreased memory, depression, and dependency to inappropriate behavior and sexual disinterest or preoccupation (Mauss-Clum & Ryan, 1981). The wife may feel all alone with her problems, since the brain-injured husband may appear quite normal to the casual observer. Yet she needs to mourn the specific losses that her mate has experienced, as well as the loss (without death) of the person she married. Yet the mourning process is compromised because she cannot openly mourn his "death" (Ziegler, 1987). The healthy spouse may experience a feeling of entrapment. If she contemplates leaving the marriage, she may realize that there would be no one to care for her husband. Guilt feelings arise and are reinforced by the expectations of others. Therapy may be the only safe place for such feelings to be safely expressed. And if she chooses to stay in the role of caretaker, her efforts will not always be welcomed, since her husband may respond with resentment at being "parented."

17.3.1. Healthy versus Pathological Mourning

If a "loved one" of a patient in psychotherapy has a terminal illness, the therapy patient may enter into a period of anticipatory mourning, which may include discussing the possibility of the loved one's dying and grieving in anticipation of such a loss. The therapy patient may want to talk about funeral preparations or other arrangements for after the death, or may be concerned about how to discuss the impending death with the terminally ill patient. There may also be ambivalence about the person's possible death, and, if the sick person lingers for a long time or actually survives, other emotions, such as guilt and anger, may surface.

If the loved one dies, a degree of emotional detachment may be evident. It is not unusual for the relatives of persons who have died to avoid direct discussions about the deceased in the months following the loss (Rando, 1983). This is a way of coping by distancing themselves from the death.

Coping with the actual death of a significant other raises the question of what constitutes healthy or nonpathological mourning. The *Diagnostic and Statistical Manual of Mental Disorders* (DSM-III; American Psychiatric Association, 1980) describes uncomplicated bereavement as lasting about two months, and suggests that symptoms such as depression persisting after that time could be pathological. This is a much shorter time than that reported in the literature or observed clinically (Koocher, 1986). Adaptation to loss occurs gradually and over an extended period of time, and symptoms of grief may be triggered years following the death of a loved one.

17.3.2. The Working-Through Process

The death of a family member produces significant repercussions in the family network. And years after, certain family members may obsess over their own actions during the course of the illness. For example, in many circumstances a sick family member may not be well enough or mentally competent enough to make decisions about his or her own treatment. Thus, the physician presents the options to the family. Later, after the person's death, the family not only mourns the loss but also must deal with the repercussions of the decisions made. There is the guilt for having hastened the death by going along with the choice to discontinue life-support systems, or the guilt for having opted for heroic measures, only to watch the loved one live for months, but suffering terribly. "I thought I was doing the right thing for my mother," a woman lamented, years after her own mother's death from a brain tumor. "They told me that chemo might give her another six months. I didn't know what to do. They left all the decisions to me. Maybe I was being selfish; I didn't want her to die. Just to have her with me for even a few more months seemed worth it. I didn't realize that the side effects would be so horrible. I never meant to make her suffer. I never should have let them treat her anymore."

18

Research Methodology: A Critique

The research in psychotherapy has been plagued by methodological problems. In all fairness to the researchers, it is not easy to conduct rigorous studies with human subjects. Standards may need to be compromised by ethical and legal considerations. And practical problems interfere with getting adequate samples or reliable and valid measures of successful treatment.

The current literature is a mix of clinical reports, anecdotes, case studies, and subjective impressions, with few well-controlled empirical studies (Burish & Lyles, 1983). Most of the research suffers from small, and not representative samples, inadequate control groups, and dependent measures that are unreliable and, in some cases, of questionable validity. Differences in outcome may arise if the research design is longitudinal (following the same patients over time), or cross-sectional (comparing different groups of subjects at different stages of the disease).

18.1. Operational Definitions and Mediating Variables

The same illness may be defined in different ways (e.g., pain, headache, or blood pressure rating), with each study using its own set of operational definitions. Measures of the dependent variable (e.g., depression, attitude, physical symptoms) may be based on medical records, examiner ratings or interviews, or patient self-reports—each having its own bias.

Those administering treatment, particularly psychological interventions, may have quite different orientations and a wide variety of training (e.g., nurses, physicians, psychologists), which could influence the type and quality of treatment and the eventual outcome. For example, studies reporting that psychological counseling has little or no effect are often based on short-term interventions, with those engaged in the psychological treatment providing counseling rather than the more in-depth therapy required to deal with deep-seated fears and anxieties. On the other side, reported treatment effects may not endure over time, and most studies lack long-term follow-up assessment of patient functioning.

Since medication plays a role in affecting mood, pain, and sexual dysfunction, its effects need to be controlled or studied as part of the research. Practically and ethically, it is difficult to control for differences in type and amount of medication. However, Binik (1983) suggests (a) using dosage as a covariate, (b) comparing groups taking specific medications with those not taking them, or (c) comparing patients before, during, and after taking certain drugs.

Contradictory findings about the extent of depression or other emotional reactions may be related to the scale used to measure affect. For example, the Minnesota Multiphasic Personality Inventory (MMPI) is often used to assess emotional responses to illness, particularly the scales Hs (Hypochondriacal), D (Depressed), and Hy (Hysterical). Many of the items on these scales ask people to confirm or deny statements about their health, such as "I am about as able to work as I ever was." "I am in just as good physical health as most of my friends." "During the past few years I have been well most of the time."

A physically ill patient who admits to poor health is not necessarily clinically depressed or suffering from a character disorder, as some scales might suggest. Thus, high scores on the MMPI, for example, may reflect real symptoms related to the physical illness (e.g., pain, inability to sleep, lack of energy), rather than the psychopathology the instrument was designed to identify (Prokop & Bradley, 1981; Watson & Kendall, 1983). When inventories are used that do not rely so heavily on somatic items (e.g., the Dempsey Depression Scale, or the California Psychological Inventory), the extent of emotional problems reported is often not as great (Freidenbergs *et al.*, 1981–1982).

18.2. SAMPLING PROBLEMS

There are many practical problems in getting large representative samples. For one, it is difficult to get large numbers of patients who have the same disease and are undergoing the same treatment. Also, patients studied may not be homogeneous even if they do have the same disease. They may differ on medical variables found to have important effects on outcome: severity of the illness, duration, site of the illness, and time since treatment (Gordon *et al.*, 1980). They may also differ on important demographic variables, such as socioeconomic level, ethnicity, sex, age, educational level—factors associated with the number of physical symptoms and stress (Cronkite & Moos, 1984). And patients may vary in terms of the physical and emotional status prior to the illness and treatment.

The setting may pose a bias as well. Hospitals, for example, treat different types of patients. Those seen in private university hospital settings, where the sample size can be large, may not be the same as those seen in public hospitals or private practice. And those in inpatient wards differ from those in outpatient wards in terms of variables such as severity of illness and environmental stress. Thus, samples may not be representative, coming from quite different patient populations.

18.3. CONTROL GROUPS

Often there is no control group, or when included it is inadequate. When choosing a control group, one needs to be clear about the questions that can be answered, considering the factors that can be controlled. Comparing those suffering from different physical illnesses, for example, does not enable one to tease out what is common to illness in general, such as the effects of hospitalization, or emotional reactions, such as depression. Also the groups may not be comparable in important ways—for example, severity of illness, treatment, time since occurrence, and demographic factors. Such initial differences between control and experimental groups make it difficult to explain differences that may be of interest in the study. If the general population statistic is used for comparison, there may be important factors other than illness that influence the observed differences, such as age and socioeconomic status.

A no-treatment control group is good as long as the patients are randomly assigned to treatment and control groups. This can help to control for placebo effects that may result from the attention and expectations of being treated *per se*, rather than from a particular treatment. The no-treatment group can control for the effects of time, since patients gradually adjust to their illnesses, and improvement may have little or no relationship to treatment. The patients, as well as those involved with the patients, should, insofar as possible, have no knowledge of who is in the control group and who is in the experimental group, or they may inadvertently give special attention or better ratings to one group over the other.

However, withholding potentially useful treatment from patients is considered inhumane. Yet research requires such controls to be sure it is the treatment and not other factors causing the effect. The argument is made that in the long run more people will benefit by a well-run study than will be hurt by being in the control group and not getting care. Of course, this is of little consolation to those in the control group. A compromise approach is that which occurred when testing the prophylactic effects of aspirin on heart attack (Steering Committee on the Physician's Health Study Research Group, 1988). When the positive effect became so strongly evident during the course of the research, the study was terminated so all patients could benefit from the experience.

18.4. CONCLUSIONS

In summary, the results of research are useful for those working with the medically ill because it helps them to understand what is to be expected and what may be unusual responses. Because of the methodological limitations (and sometimes the overzealousness of the researchers, who believe so much in their own theories and treatments), the actual evidence may not be as strong as reported. Small samples (sometimes only one patient), inadequate control groups, and low correlations are only a few of the limitations that caution against generalizing the results to others. Through the use of computers and more sophisticated statistical techniques, such as meta-analysis, studies are emerging that allow practitioners to apply the results with more confidence. Although research in health psychology has its limitations, it is still useful in pointing out trends and cautioning about misconceptions. And despite the generalizations that can be made when studying groups, individuals still have their own unique ways of responding and their special ways of being.

V

Case Studies of Specific Illnesses: Psychodynamic Issues

Introduction

The case studies illustrate the psychodynamic issues that arise when a person is faced with particular medical conditions. The cases reveal how characterological makeup, developmental issues, internal conflicts, and interpersonal relationships get played out in the course of therapy with the physically ill. Brief discussions of each disease are included as background to aid the nonmedical therapist. To protect the patients' identities, names and some facts have been changed.

Case 1

From the Diary of a
Thirteen-Year-Old (Asthma)

1.1. MAGGIE

Breath. Everyone takes breath for granted. But you, you're an asthmatic person suffering one of your worst attacks. A slight drizzle earlier in the evening was all you needed for a start. The extremely warm September night doesn't help either. The people around see you sitting there nervous and shaking, and the perspiration rolling down your face and neck.

Your chest feels tight as though your windpipe had been squeezed into half its size. Your lungs are tired and seem as though they're ready to burst. With each deep and painful breath you think only of relief. Pills, pills. You've taken pills, but they tend only to make you more nervous. You feel nauseated, but can get no relief. Every breath seems to be the last. You think of your friends and how they wanted you to be with them tonight. But you had to refuse—because of asthma. They didn't understand, because you were right there talking to them. They didn't realize every word spoken and every short breath was agony. You put up a big front for them, but after they had gone you went back to the treatments: pills, atomizers, hot tea.

Now you're alone in your bedroom. Everyone in the house is asleep. But no, not you. You're an asthmatic patient, remember. Oh yes, you remember—with every gasp, with every wheeze. To lie down would be more torture. Again you feel nauseated. The sweat rolls down your face. You pity yourself but at last you've given in. Yes, there is a way to get relief and that night's sleep you've been dreaming of. A shot. [Referring to the injections that her parents can administer.] The needle won't even hurt, because you know in one minute relief will come. Your breath will be regular again. Your chest will feel hollow and light, but you don't care. A nervous feeling comes over you as you would imagine to be the same feeling a dope addict gets from a narcotic. Only of course in a simplified version. Yes, you'll take that shot and thank God for taking care of you and understanding.

Maggie wrote this entry in her diary one hot August night, sitting all alone in her room. She had had her first asthma attack when she was 2 years old. Her only memory was of lying in the backseat of the family car, looking

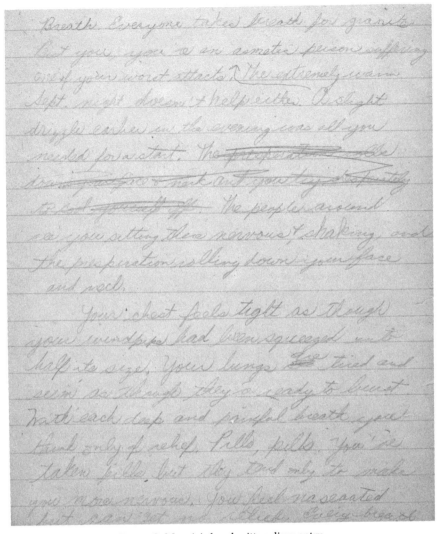

FIGURE 2. Maggie's handwritten diary entry.

at the bright red flames of the steel mills' coke ovens in the distance, and not being able to get her breath. She was one of the lucky ones, however. Her condition, although with her over the years, only flared up once in a while, mostly during ragweed season at the end of August. When she was quite small, she would occasionally feign an attack following a bad dream, to get her mother to come into her room during the night to comfort her. But most of the time, she was like any other little girl, except she kept hearing the cautions in her head: "Don't run too much or you'll get short of breath." "Stay out of the weeds when you play." Even too much laughing could bring on an attack. When she went to high school she was told: "If you want to be in the marching band, play a percussion instrument, not one you have to blow." And forget it, those summer hayrides were like death.

She kept her condition a secret from most of her friends, and those who did know didn't understand anyway. Sometimes, as she got older and stayed out later in the damp evening air, she would hardly be able to catch her breath, becoming more quiet and subdued. The inside of her mouth would become ulcerated as she sucked the inside of her cheek, pulling the flesh between her teeth—a trick she had developed to feel in control, while concentrating on her regular shallow breathing.

Maggie has since grown into adulthood and has learned to avoid most of the stimuli (e.g., pollen, dust) that can trigger an attack. Although now she may have only three or four minor attacks a year, she still carries her asthma pills with her wherever she goes. The fear of being caught without them and not being able to breathe terrifies her. She also carries with her some emotional baggage: a certain overconcern with her health, and a particularly strong desire for fresh air.

1.2. ASTHMA: SOME BACKGROUND

As Maggie wrote, breathing is taken for granted by most individuals, but many patients with respiratory disease have known periods where they were unable to get their breath for considerable periods of time. The feeling has been described as suffocating, strangling, or drowning and can be very frightening.

Maggie's description of her asthmatic attack illustrates all asthmatics' hypervigilance in relation to their bodies. There can be an obsession with the nuances of breathing, and with medication and treatment. There is the fear of becoming addicted to the medication, of becoming a dope addict, because the need for relief is so great.

About 5% of Americans are affected by bronchial asthma. Muscle spasms, thick, mucous secretions, and tissue swelling serve to narrow the bronchial tubes, sometimes for days, obstructing air exchange to the lungs (Friedman & Booth-Kewley, 1987). Reactions are often caused by allergies (e.g., pollen, dust, animal dandruff). For some the condition is seasonal or sporadic, depending upon their contact with triggering agents. For others the condition may be chronic or so severe that hospitalization is required.

Asthmatics often suffer from other allergic conditions, such as eczema, allergic rhinitis, and food allergies. This suggests that these individuals are hypersensitive to agents in their environment, with their bodies rejecting certain substances that for others are not a problem. Thus, asthma is no longer considered strictly an allergic reaction or a psychological response to stress. It is now recognized that physical, immunological, and psychological factors all have their roles to play.

1.2.1. Psychological Reactions

Some of the earliest attempts to explain the cause of asthma made use of psychosomatic theories. Most of these theories, however, were based extensively on clinical impressions, and evidence supporting them is quite weak (Creer, 1978; Friedman & Booth-Kewley, 1987; Weiner, 1977). Some of the theories posited that aggressive, dependent, and anxious persons were more prone to asthmatic attacks. The psychological origin was thought to be strong unconscious dependency wishes toward the mother, along with fear of separation. Although individual case studies may support this theory, it has not held up under rigorous scientific scrutiny (Thompson & Thompson, 1985).

Creer (1982), in a summary of the literature on the psychological factors in asthma, notes that there is little evidence to suggest that children with asthma have disturbed relationships with their mothers. Studies that have followed asthmatics longitudinally over a period of years yield data that indicate that asthmatic children seem to develop in an age-appropriate and developmentally appropriate manner. In individual cases, maladaptive behaviors may develop as a response to the illness. Creer concluded that there is no unique personality type specifically associated with asthma, and that claims that asthmatic attacks occur as a result of failure to fully express emotions, such as anger, have not been supported by objective research.

It is not disputed, however, that emotional states can be associated with asthma attacks. In some cases, psychological factors, such as stress or anxiety, trigger the condition, and emotional upsets can play a role in maintaining the asthmatic symptoms once they have been triggered. But which comes first, the condition or the emotional reactions? It is not surprising that those susceptible to asthma might be more anxious, dependent or fearful. Also, once an attack starts, the person naturally becomes upset, and the physiological reactions of the upset may further exacerbate the asthmatic symptoms.

Some have speculated that asthmatic breathing is a learned response, in the classical Pavlovian sense (Thompson & Thompson, 1985). At first there is a response to an allergen; then certain stimuli that the individual has learned to associate with an attack eventually become conditioned stimuli for an actual attack.

1.2.1.1. Personal and Interpersonal Reactions

Depression during or between attacks may be related to a lowered self-image or to an inability to participate in interpersonal relationships to the fullest. The fact that this is a hidden illness, where the symptoms are not obvious, can present problems because people do not realize, or may forget, that the patient is not feeling well, and thus they may make unrealistic demands.

The restrictions in the life-style and "feeling different" can be particularly difficult for children and adolescents. If they are being treated with corticosteroids, physical changes may occur that affect self-image and sexuality: obesity, acne, hirsutism (hair growth on face or body), and easy bruising. And depression may arise from the hovering, underlying fear of impending death (Thompson & Thompson, 1985). During an asthma attack a patient may feel panicky or fearful of dying. Some are haunted throughout life by this fear. They may become increasingly anxious that they will be caught unawares and not be prepared for an attack (i.e., not have their medication with them). Thus, they may limit their activities and life-styles.

Labeling asthma as a "psychosomatic illness" adds additional stress. Psychosomatic popularly implies not simply an interaction between physical and emotional but a psychological cause for the disorder. This puts an added burden on the sufferer, who now feels responsible for causing the illness, and guilty for the strain and disruption it causes in the patient's family. Others may see asthmatics as "neurotic," may believe that the illness is all in their heads, that if they could control their moods or emotions, they wouldn't have the symptoms. Thus, there may be little sympathy or understanding, and, in fact, there may be irritation at the patient for being ill.

1.2.2. Behavioral Management and Secondary Gain

Patients may derive secondary gain from having asthma and may use their symptoms in a manipulative way. The theory of operant conditioning is helpful in understanding how symptom formation may shape family responses to an illness such as asthma. For example, an asthma attack may be followed by increased attention, affection, and support, responses that are highly reinforcing. The patient may learn that the symptoms serve to protect against unpleasant or negative experiences, such as going to work or school, or facing the anger or criticism of others.

Stoudemire (1985) suggest that these learned maladaptive responses may explain why, in some cases, young patients show temporary improvement when separated from their parents.

Although behavior management of the physical symptoms of asthma has not been encouraging, behavioral and educational strategies have been useful in diminishing maladaptive behaviors, such as noncompliance, malingering, and deliberate provocation of attacks (Stoudemire, 1985). Psychodynamic interventions can also be of help in relieving the person's depression, sense of helplessness, self-image concerns, and feelings of guilt.

Case 2

Reemergence of the Repressed (Postpolio)

2.1. ELISE

Elise was one of those unfortunate enough to have contracted polio during the epidemic in the early 1950s. She was fortunate, however, that she was left with no obvious disability, except some muscle weakness. Now, 30 years later, at the age of 43, Elise began to experience increasing muscle weakness, pain in her joints, and a general aching in her body, not unlike the flu. The polio had left her with a mild scoliosis, and the weakening muscles were unable to prevent the gradually increasing curvature of the spine that threatened to crush her heart and lungs.

Elise consulted a top specialist and consented to an extensive back operation, with the expectation that with bone fusion she would be able to stand straight and resume her normal life. No one had expected the complications that would follow the surgery, that would leave her too weak to go without the brace, crush her hope, and devastate her psychologically. Instead of being a solution, the surgery was only the beginning of years of misery. The spine did not fuse completely, and the previously weakened muscles, even further weakened by the surgery, could not support the back as well as had been hoped. Over a two-year period, Elise had three major back surgeries. Still she found herself in the unwanted brace, unable to lead what she felt was a normal life.

The brace became the symbol of her helplessness. When she was a child with polio, her own inner determination, supported by her mother's excessive use of denial, kept her fighting to be as normal as possible, giving up the brace as soon as she could, and before the physicians of the day thought she should. Now she feared becoming severely handicapped.

After the first operation failed, Elise began to mistrust the physician. "Doctors should be more aware that they often destroy people instead of help them," she would later say. "They are like carpenters. They come in, do the job, and are finished." She felt the surgeon had "screwed up," that he had minimized the problem, that he had lied to her. With each approaching appointment to his office, she would become overwhelmed with anxiety and would question and challenge him relentlessly. He responded defensively by being evasive and curt. Despite his recognized expertise in his field, she had come to realize that he had little experience with polio patients, and his usual techniques did not work well with her.

Elise began to mistrust him after the first surgery did not work as well as had been expected. The surgeon misperceived the basis of her anger and what he saw as resistance to further treatment (although she did eventually undergo two additional surgeries). He himself may have felt bad that he had failed this woman. But he further alienated her by avoiding answering her questions or giving her information. He undoubtedly was afraid of a lawsuit in this litigious day and age. He was also unaware that previously repressed memories of her childhood experience in hospitals and convalescent homes were now coming to the fore, unleashing powerful emotions. Elise herself was confused by the extent and uncontrollable nature of her reactions.

Adding to Elise's anxieties were the articles she had been reading about the "postpolio syndrome" (i.e., the aftereffects of polio that appear many years later). Although learning about her condition had helped her understand what was happening to her (and also helped her to educate her physicians), the information about the potentially deteriorating course of the condition was extremely upsetting. The fact that research was under way gave her little consolation, since she felt she would be too old to benefit. She obsessed about the "quality of life" and thought about suicide as a possible solution. She did not want to become a burden to others, nor did she want to become totally incapacitated and dependent. One of the physicians involved in her treatment, sensing her deep depression, referred her for psychotherapy.

In therapy, Elise recalled the first week of her polio attack, before it had been diagnosed: the high fever, the delirium, the muscle weakness, and the terrible fear that maybe she would never walk again. Now she knew this fear again; it seemed all too familiar and just as strong. Overlapping themes appeared: distrust of authority, feelings of abandonment, guilt at having caused her own condition, guilt over the repressed anger at her mother whose denial of her illness delayed her being taken to the hospital for several weeks. (The failure of parents to recognize the seriousness of the child's illness was not atypical, as revealed in the early research on polio in families—Davis, 1963.)

When Elise was hospitalized, no one talked to her directly. She was an adolescent. Physicians would deal only with her parents, or would speak about her to each other in front of her or in nearby hallways, as though she were not there—yet she could overhear everything they were saying. She was 13, intelligent, and angry that these adults did not treat her as a person.

And she was scared. She never knew what was to happen to her. She pieced together what she overheard, trying to understand, trying to gain some control over her young life. She began to mistrust those who had authority over her, feeling manipulated and lied to. She was told she would be home in three months, only to be kept for nine. Had they lied or had they just neglected to include her in their discussions of her treatment? Frightened and feeling abandoned by parents whom she perceived as having relinquished their own protective power and who rarely visited her, she began to act out: resisting treatment, crying, arguing. To her memory, these desperate attempts for attention and control were only met by threats and anger from the staff. Elise had felt that no one understood what she was going through.

Under the tenets of the treatment methods of that time, she exercised as much as possible, so by age 15 she was no longer in a convalescent home or in need of any supports or prosthetic devices. Elise could "pass." No one would need to know that she had had polio, something her mother had been very concerned about. Her mother had felt very guilty and embarrassed about her daughter's having polio. She felt that the disease was a disgrace and a social stigma, and although the resulting disability was minimal, she harbored fears that no one would marry her daughter because of the polio. As a full-grown woman, Elise continued to keep the secret, telling only immediate family and a few close friends. With the new symptoms, however, it was becoming harder and harder to keep the secret close to home.

Elise married young and had two children, despite warnings from her obstetrician, who feared she could not carry them to term because of her polio-weakened stomach muscles. Years later, one child was hyperactive and diagnosed as learning-disabled, something that caused Elise great feelings of guilt because she secretly felt that her polio had somehow affected her child. Nevertheless, Elise was an active mother and a devoted homemaker. She became an excellent skier and swimmer and loved to bicycle. She enjoyed driving in her suburban community, and she had a sense of independence and control in her life.

Now there was also her anger at her increasing dependency, which conflicted with her need to be taken care of. And the ramifications of this conflict were increasingly felt at home. Even sedentary activities were barely possible, since anxiety and depression interfered with her concentration. And she could not reduce her tension through her favorite sports. She became dependent on her husband, Jim, since she could no longer drive to the store, to the beauty parlor, to see friends. She was dependent upon him around the house as well because she had difficulty bending or lifting even moderately heavy objects. The frustration and the dependency increasingly resulted in angry outbursts at her husband.

Jim, not unexpectedly, began showing signs of the strain. He dealt with his frustrations through his customary defenses of repressions and withdrawal. Attempts to put on a cheerful front were only temporarily helpful. Her fear and despair became his. He worried about her future, about the quality of her medical care, about her desire to take risks, to do things now while she still could. He worried about her emotional well-being, since he sensed the depth of her depression. In effect, he became her "superego," cautioning her, trying to help her to be rational in a situation in which reliable information was lacking, a sitution fraught with emotion. Needless to say, if one carries the Freudian analogy further, her "id" rebelled against his protective attempts.

Elise seemed to find support in psychotherapy. It was extremely difficult for her to talk about her earlier experiences with polio and the convalescence. She felt that all that had gone on before should have been resolved, and she was disturbed at what she saw as a personal weakness that these earlier experiences were still a live issue for her. In therapy she could talk about her fears and her frustrations about her compromised quality of life. With many postpolio patients, the extent of their symptoms is not obvious to others, and they try as before "to do what others do." Expectations, both physically and emotionally, may be high, as family and friends forget or try to get the patient to forget the ever-present fear of the future.

Elise continues in therapy, using it as supportive therapy as new physical problems arise, and for insight as deep-seated unresolved emotional issues surface.

2.2. POSTPOLIO SYNDROME

Polio survivors in the United States are estimated to number between 200,000 and 300,000 (Laurie, 1980; Laurie, Maynard, Fischer, & Raymond, 1984; Roosevelt Warm Springs Institute for Rehabilitation, 1982, 1983). At least 132,000 of these people were struck with the disease during the 1952–1954 epidemic. Now, decades later, many who felt they had overcome the illness and made their adjustments are beginning to experience increasing weakness and pain, the cause of which is yet to be fully understood (Halstead & Wiechers, 1985; 1987; Laurie, 1980; National Institute of Handicapped Research, 1986; Roosevelt Warm Springs Institute for Rehabilitation, 1982, 1983).

From 20 to 50% of polio survivors over 40 years of age are reported as exhibiting latent effects; it is expected that the percentage will increase as the population ages and physicians become more astute in their diagnosis (Halstead & Wiechers, 1985, 1987; Horowitz, 1985; Laurie, 1980; Laurie *et al.*, 1984). A paradoxical effect of the success of the polio vaccines is that there are few physicians today who have training or experience treating polio patients. Most health care providers are unaware of the condition, and patients, frustrated and scared, must search for help. Misdiagnosis is not uncommon.

As the extent and nature of the original disabilities vary, so do these later symptoms. Those with limited breathing reserve may now need mechanical assistance. Patients with even minor deformities or weakness of spine or limb may develop painful degenerative joint disease or nerve compression, as a result of continuous weight bearing on the joints from everyday activities. Weakened back muscles may result in severe scoliosis, necessitating surgery. Some who were able to walk without any auxiliary devices now find themselves having to use crutches or a brace; others may need a wheelchair. Persons who have been using wheelchairs, but who had the use of their hands and arms, may now experience a loss of function. After years of being independent, some find themselves depending on others to feed them; mouth sticks or other such devices may be needed to perform routine tasks at home and on the job.

2.2.1. Psychological Resistance/Distrust of Authority

Compounding the situation is that recommendations given years ago (e.g., to exercise as much as possible) may have contributed to the present condition. Today these same patients are being told to take it easy and to rest, not to exert themselves, to accept their lessening of strength and stamina. Resistance develops, since these recommendations often involve curtailing many pleasures and becoming more dependent upon others. Patients realize that recent prescriptions are based on new untested theories, as were many of the contradictory prescriptions given years ago. Thus, health care providers find patients avoiding treatment, minimizing their conditions, disregarding advice—in effect, not wanting to become less active and more dependent, particularly when, to their minds, no one is really sure. For those who had milder cases of the disease, who had not thought of themselves as disabled, the new weakness and pain shakes their sense of self. The unknown course of the disease makes it even more difficult to make adjustments, since they do not know what they are going to be expected to adjust to.

2.2.2. The Emotional Components

Postpolio patients now experience, both physically and emotionally, a recurrence of the disabling disease (Backman, 1987; Kohl, 1987). The weakness, the pain, the fear of never being able to walk are reminiscent of the earlier episode, causing the patients to relive much of the overwhelming emotional feelings that had been repressed (Frick & Bruno, 1986). Their feelings are not unlike those of stroke patients when dealing with crises in their illness (Bucher *et al.*, 1984), or cancer patients who experience a recurrence of the disease (Koocher, 1986; Koocher & O'Malley, 1981).

As most postpolio patients were children or adolescents when they struggled with polio and its aftermath, many of the needs and behaviors that appear under the new stressful situation are reflective of unresolved childhood issues (Bozarth, 1987; Davis, 1963). Fears of being restricted and trapped, of being abandoned, emanating from the previous experience in hospitals and convalescent homes, reemerge. Returning to the use of a brace or wheelchair, after having struggled to overcome the need for such aids 25 or 30 years before, may activate long-standing emotional conflicts, many of which center around issues of dependency. Resistance to being put in a brace may appear unrealistic to the physician and the family, if physical support is now needed, but this resistance may be an expression of the person's fear of impending lack of mobility.

Patients' complaints about not being able to swim, bicycle, or walk for any length of time may seem self-indulgent or unrealistic to others, but what needs to be understood is that these are expressions of fear of what is to come: fear of not being able to walk or breathe. Complaints about no longer being able to drive, for example, may be expressions of anxiety related to dependency and lack of control in one's life. Other psychological issues, such as grieving for loss of function and loss of former identity and sense of self, social withdrawal, and depression, may also be present.

Case 3

The Lonely Road (Prostate Cancer)

3.1. HOWARD

Howard was referred for psychotherapy by his treating physician because he was severely depressed. Tears would well up in his eyes during examinations, and he was unable to speak without crying. The idea of seeing a psychotherapist bothered him because he saw it as a further recognition that he was losing control of his life. He eventually agreed to go into therapy, however, since it was becoming clearer to him that he could no longer cope on his own. And "on his own" was how he felt, despite the fact that he had a wife and a stepson.

Howard, now 50, had been working for an insurance company. He had worked his way up to a good position and had had a fairly comfortable life. His first wife had died of cancer about eight years previously. He found it difficult to speak of her. That life seemed far away now, and the memories of her only added to his fears since he learned of his own diagnosis: prostate cancer. He had three children by that marriage, now all grown and into their own lives, living in different parts of the country.

Howard had met Catherine, his present wife, about three years after he had been widowed. Catherine, a successful businesswoman, seemed to have the strength and direction that he needed. And her husband coincidentally had died of cancer. She too was looking for solace and companionship. Howard and Catherine married, and with her two young boys, they moved into Howard's home to start a life together. But they only had "two good years."

Howard began to notice that he urinated more often than usual; in fact, it reached the point where no sooner would he fall asleep than he would be up running to the bathroom again. During the day he was totally fatigued and was becoming snappish at home and in the office. He had noticed some pains in the pelvic area but tried to ignore these. However, the day he noticed blood in his urine he knew he had to see his doctor. That was three years ago.

3.1.1. Psychotherapy

When Howard came to his first psychotherapy session, he was like a man without emotion, speaking in a monotone. Yet the tears in his eyes betrayed the torment he felt. He had been told that his cancer had metastasized to his bones. He was afraid of the future, of becoming an invalid. He was aware that he was getting progressively weaker. He was troubled with severe headaches and back pain. The medication he took for the pain left him numb and disoriented. His first wife had suffered terribly for six months. He didn't want to go through what she had gone through.

By the second session, Howard was able to speak more freely about his thoughts of death and dying. He felt he was just marking time. He said he was prepared to die but wished he could know how much time he had, what the course of the disease would be, and what the end would be like. He spoke of suicide as an option, but even in his current distress he said he was not ready to end his life—maybe if he were really suffering—but not now.

Howard had had several operations, including an orchiectomy (removal of the testes). Impotency is one of the unfortunate side effects of this surgery, and Howard was not spared. Not that his sex life had been any too great before the operation. The fatigue and depression from the illness had severely reduced his desire early on, and his wife's own difficulties, having to deal once more with a terminally ill husband, had caused her to pull away even before the operation.

Howard felt like a shell of a man. His former identity had all but been taken from him. Sexually he described himself as a eunuch. But sex didn't seem all that important anymore. His life was taken up with treatments, appointments with doctors, keeping track of medication, and just getting around. He moved very slowly, both walking and sitting were painful, and the headaches made it difficult to concentrate. Howard did continue to go to the office once a week. Although a colleague was filling in for him, he would turn up for a few hours, open his mail, and visit with his fellow workers.

When he had time, he tried desperately to keep track of his health insurance. Which form to submit for which bills? What had been paid? Reimbursed? Who would keep it all in order, should he become even more incapacitated? But keeping some order and control in his life was important. And he was glad to have the extensive insurance coverage.

Time spent walking around the streets and sitting on park benches was filled with conflict. He had been raised to feel that people worked, that you were to be productive. He had had little compassion for those on unemployment or welfare. He felt that they could work somehow if they wanted to. Now, at age 50, he found himself sharing park benches with senior citizens, and walking slowly, almost with a shuffle, supported by a cane. He was not an elegant sight. On rainy days he stayed home.

Howard's psychotherapy was at an outpatient clinic in a hospital. The psychotherapist raised the possibility of his doing volunteer work in the hospital. Howard was quite agreeable. The therapist made arrangements for him to be involved in remedial training and possibly computer training in the hospital's rehabilitation program. But Howard never had the chance to try. Each time he was to begin, he had to cancel because of a complication with his illness. Eventually, he just gave up the idea of working.

3.1.1.1. Frustrations with the Medical World

One of Howard's issues in therapy was his frustration with the medical profession. Like many so afflicted, he went from doctor to doctor, hospital to hospital, looking for one who could help. Eventually, Howard settled on a well-known oncologist to handle his chemotherapy. However, he came to find Dr. J unapproachable and cold. Howard tried to tell himself that the physician's expertise was more important than his bedside manner. But the frustrations and the accompanying angers bubbled under the surface.

The conflicts came to a head when Dr. J became ill and had his associate take over the case. Dr. S, the new physician, was not able to deal with Howard's need for human contact and was brusque in their interactions. During a hospitalization, Howard was left to lie in bed for three days awaiting the visit of another specialist. The days dragged on. Dr. S was nowhere in sight, nor was the specialist. Howard verbally flailed at the nurses and was considered ''a difficult patient''—which indeed he had become. Eventually, he checked himself out.

Through a personal friend he found another oncologist who, though less well known, had a more relaxed and personable manner. Howard become more relaxed as well, and even his health seemed to improve, at least for a time. He had opted to risk a bit of professional ''excellence'' in order to have a more complete relationship with his physician.

3.1.1.2. The Growing Need for Care

Howard's emotional needs increased as his condition worsened. Even before his illness he was somewhat self-centered and taking care of his dying wife had been a strain. He loved her, yet busied himself at the office, never missing a day of work until the very end. But he did see that she had round-the-clock nurses. Now, as he faced his own illness, feelings of guilt crept over him.

His current regression put strains on his relationship with Catherine, his present wife. He felt that she was really not there for him and resented her efforts to continue with her own life, going to work, seeing friends, and taking care of her children. She rarely accompanied him on his medical visits, leaving him to make his own way slowly to and from taxis and through the large halls of the medical centers. People stared at him shuffling along, but his determination kept help at bay. He was terrified of falling, as he had more than once at home.

Catherine and Howard occasionally did go out socially, sometimes for dinner, but he had no appetite. And trying to make conversation with acquaintances was difficult. At the same time, Howard resented friends' pulling away, and he could enumerate all those who no longer called.

His need for attention put him in direct competition with his stepsons, upon whom his wife now concentrated more and more. The tensions erupted into constant fighting over "your children" and "my children," with Catherine attacking the behavior of Howard's adult children. Why weren't they more involved in his care? To her, their few phone calls and occasional visits did not make up for their obvious distance, both physical and emotional.

Howard could not bear the angry criticism, and as tensions mounted he felt a closer and closer bond with his former family. A sister in Arizona had asked him to come to stay with her. He felt too young to go out there with all those old retired people. Yet the sun would feel good, and he was dreading the oncoming winter. But moving would effectively mean the end of his marriage. His wife's life was her career and her children. They were rooted in the East. He no longer fit into their routine.

3.1.1.3. Family Therapy

For a time Howard resisted the idea of couples therapy. True, on those nights when he woke up crying in pain, Catherine was there by his side, comforting him, helping him to take his pain medication. But in the morning he was alone again. He was torn between gratitude and despair. Perhaps there was something to salvage. He asked Catherine to come to a joint therapy session. She refused; she was too busy; it would mean taking time off from work.

Then one day Catherine agreed to see the therapist, but she wanted to do so the first time alone. She was having problems with her eldest son and needed some advice. So an appointment was arranged. Catherine was a somewhat plump, attractive middle-aged woman, well kept in her business suit. Keeping in control was her issue: no show of emotion, telling the therapist that she was only there to get help for her son. No, the marriage was not a problem. The boy, David, was 16 years old and having severe problems in school. His grades were dropping and this week he had had a fight with a classmate, breaking his glasses. The school's guidance counselor had expressed concern and recommended professional help.

From a family therapy perspective, her son's acting-out might signal his call for help for a family disintegrating before his young eyes. Although his own motives were probably not conscious, his acting-out might have been a way to get his parents close together again, to function as a unit while they were trying to help him, or to get help for themselves as part of his treatment.

The therapist concurred with Catherine that her son did need help; however, Catherine was firm that family therapy was out of the question. She would have no time, and according to her the problem had nothing to do with her and Howard. Yes, the boys knew of Howard's condition, but not how severe it was. Yes, they were quietly attached to him; he was the only father they really remembered. Whether they overheard his painful night awakenings, or observed his deterioration, she could not say. It was never mentioned. Denial was everywhere. Catherine's focus was on her children. She had had one husband die and now was determined not to let this other man pull her down with him. She was trying desperately to maintain control as her own world started falling apart again.

Individual therapy with children was not part of the outpatient services of the hospital clinic, except as a part of family therapy. Catherine said she preferred an adolescent specialist for David, and was given an outside referral. A week later she called to say she had found someone else through her own network.

3.1.1.4. Termination Phase

Howard continued to come for his twice-weekly appointments. He was disappointed that Catherine had not wanted to meet with him to discuss their mutual concerns, but he was not surprised. Her children were all she cared about. They were her family, not him. As the months passed, Howard began having double vision and more headaches. A tumor had been discovered in the right side of his brain. Remarkably, after several weeks of radiation, the symptoms disappeared. He weathered that period quite well. But it was another indication that the cancer had metastasized.

With winter approaching he flew to Arizona to find a place to live. His sister wanted him to be in her house, but he wanted to be on his own, at least as long as he could. He thought about buying a new car. He had always wanted a Porsche. But his legs felt weak, and he wasn't as alert as he felt he should be. And the doctor had said no driving. Howard came back from Arizona after a few weeks with a small but thoughtful gift for the therapist. Although he came to therapy a couple of times after that, he missed the next scheduled appointments. When the therapist telephoned, he was confused and could not figure out who was on the other end. A month later he went back to Arizona.

3.2. Prostate Cancer

Cancer of the prostate accounts for almost 20% of cancers in males, second only to lung cancer (American Cancer Society, 1986). The condition is rare in those under 55, with 70 being the average age (National Cancer Institute, 1981). The rates are higher among blacks than whites, and more married men than single men develop it (American Cancer Society, 1981).

The prostate is a gland about the size of a chestnut. It lies just below the urinary bladder and surrounds the first inch of the urethra, a canal that carries urine from the bladder. The secretion of the prostate provides part of the fluid for ejaculation.

Cancer of the prostate usually involves enlargement of the gland, which then obstructs the urethra. The signs and symptoms of prostatic cancer can include a variety of difficulties: weak or interrupted urine flow, frequent urination (especially at night), inability to urinate or difficulty in starting urination, urine flow that is not easily stopped, blood in the urine, painful or burning urination, and continuing pain in lower back, pelvis, or upper thighs.

The most common tumor found in the prostatic gland, however, is not malignant (i.e., not cancerous). It is called benign prostatic hypertrophy, and it afflicts about half the men in the United States over 50. Since the signs and symptoms are similar to cancer, it is important that those afflicted have regular medical examinations for a differential diagnosis. Almost all prostatic cancers begin in the part of the prostate that can be felt during a routine digital rectal examination. The only way to determine conclusively if a tumor is malignant is by biopsy. X rays and tests of the urine and blood are also conducted. These tumors are slow-growing and in the early stages may go undetected since no signs or symptoms are noticed. More than half of all prostatic cancers are caught while they are still localized; thus, yearly checkups are encouraged for those over 40. Up to 70% of patients whose tumors are localized reach the five-year survival mark, a time that is customarily used as an indication of successful treatment. For all stages of prostatic cancer combined, the five-year survival rate is over 50%.

3.2.1. Treatment and Its Aftereffects

Depending upon the stage of the cancer and the patient's age and medical history, treatment may include one or more of the following: surgery, radiation therapy, hormone treatment, and chemotherapy with anticancer drugs.

If the tumor is completely confined to the prostate, it can usually be successfully treated by surgical removal of the gland, an operation called a prostatectomy. A certain amount of nerve and tissue damage occurs, depending upon the site and extent of the surgery. In many cases there is a temporary or permanent loss of the capacity for erection and ejaculation, and in a small number of cases there may be urinary incontinence as well.

The growth of some of the cancer cells in prostate tumors is stimulated by male sex hormones. When the cancer has spread beyond the gland itself, or when there is recurrence, the testes may be surgically removed (orchiectomy), thereby eliminating a source of the hormone testosterone. Another type of hormone therapy is the administration of the female hormone estrogen. This may lead to unwanted side effects, such as breast enlargement, breast tenderness, nausea and vomiting, and water and sodium retention. Radiotherapy may be used if the cancer has spread beyond the primary site. Although the risk of impotence may be less than with surgery, gastrointestinal disturbances or bladder symptoms may result.

3.2.2. Psychological Reactions

It is not uncommon, following treatment, for patients to experience extreme distress regarding loss of function, and fears regarding attractiveness to the opposite sex. The orchiectomy in particular can be psychologically devastating, yet many men find it difficult to speak openly about their feelings, particularly those involving sexual function and masculinity. Self-doubt, depression, and anxiety may reduce the sex drive and inhibit successful adjustment (Burish & Lyles, 1983). Patients may feel exhausted because of the interrupted sleep caused by the need to urinate frequently during the night. The gastrointestinal problems, leading to intense and unexpected diarrhea, may cause inconvenience and embarrassment. Patients may limit their activities and isolate themselves from others, not wanting to share this unpleasant personal information. They may also fear these symptoms, thinking they are indications that the disease has spread rather than being the side effects of treatment. Interventions that address the psychological problems of these patients are particularly important for helping them in their journey through this often lonely and difficult ordeal.

Case 4

Anna's Dreams (Breast Cancer)

4.1. ANNA

Anna phoned her therapist from the hospital. She was very upset. She had been having disturbing dreams following her surgery, dreams that were so intense she feared she might be losing her mind. Dr. R came to the hospital as soon as she could.

Anna had been diagnosed as having breast cancer two years before. At that time she opted for a lumpectomy, which would allow her to keep her breast. After a course of chemotherapy and radiation, she gradually recovered her strength and was feeling like a winner. In less than two years, however, a tumor was discovered in the same breast. Anna was devastated. She thought they had found it all. What was the sense of having gone through those treatments? she kept asking herself. Just when she was beginning to feel better and get on with her life, the nightmare was starting all over again. And how would she know if they would get it all the second time around? This time a mastectomy was recommended. Anna also elected to have reconstructive surgery immediately thereafter.

In her dreams Anna had encountered some of her most deep-seated, primitive feelings, triggered by the recent trauma to her body and to her sense of self. These feelings terrified her. In addition, her sense of security had been shattered with the recurrence of her disease. In the dreams she experienced basic fears as she faced the unknown, alone.

4.2. Dream 1

Tanya (a friend who had also had a mastectomy) had come to the hospital with her family to smuggle Anna out. They were collecting bodies for an experiment and needed "damaged bodies." Anna remembers being with all these bodies in the dream, and "parts flying every which way." Her own body became divided in half. She had the bottom half from the waist down but could not find a top to match.

The dream was frightening. Anna was left with a feeling of helplessness. She thought she was going crazy. Although the experience of her body's being mutilated by the operation may be obvious to those hearing the dream, it was not so obvious to Anna until brought to her conscious level through dream interpretation. Unconsciously she was trying to cope with this overwhelming experience by emotionally isolating the damaged or lost part of her body from the healthy part. Through reconstructive surgery she was looking to make herself whole again. But the process was confusing and frightening.

When questioned about Tanya's role in the dream, Anna replied that Tanya had been avoiding her. She was angry with her friend for what she saw as self-centeredness in Anna's time of need. The therapist suggested that Tanya might have been avoiding Anna, consciously or unconsciously, because she could not face the possibility that she too could have a recurrence of her cancer.

4.2.1. Dream 2

Anna felt herself falling from a tall building, falling and falling and falling. She landed safely in a city, but in the middle of squalor. There was poverty and filth everywhere. She saw her old boyfriend and his children living in a very poor run-down house. Again there was a feeling of helplessness when she woke up. She still felt as if she were falling; she couldn't stop herself; her body had its own momentum and was out of her control.

In this dream Anna was an outsider looking in at what could have been. She had escaped, she had landed safely. She felt like a pioneer. She had been told that only a few thousand women had ever had breast reconstruction. Anna felt "special" to have been on this "trip" and to have survived. She admitted needing to feel special, to believe that she would be one of the ones to beat the odds.

Anna said she often had dreams about looking for a home, but never like the one she saw in this dream. The houses were usually big and beautiful, but empty. Were these dreams symbolic of her search for security, for roots? Did the house represent her own body, her empty life? She would wonder from time to time if she should have stayed with her old boyfriend. Did the squalor now represent the way she saw herself, her body, her life? Or was it what life might have been like had she stayed with him in his difficult existence? She wasn't sure.

4.2.2. Dream 3

Anna's friend Christa was very sick and upset. Anna was trying to comfort her and help her. ("Guess I'm trying to take your job," she said to the therapist when recounting the dream.) Christa wanted to get out of the hospital; she felt she had been abandoned; no one could help her. Anna reassured Christa and snuck her out.

Contrary to Anna's remark, on one level Christa represented the real Anna. Anna wanted her therapist, Dr. R, to rescue her, to comfort her, and to save her from all that she was going through. And in fact, Anna had had this dream the very night following her desperate call to Dr. R. When Dr. R asked if Anna felt she might abandon her as well, she replied, "No." She had been abandoned by the physicians. She had put her trust in them, they had treated her, yet the cancer came back. Now whom could she trust to save her life? The word *trust* came up over and over again, underlying the helplessness and lack of control that she felt.

Anna expressed relief after she and the therapist worked on the interpretation of the dreams. Dr. R suggested that the awakening of her deep-seated fears and her feelings of depersonalization were related to the trauma that she had experienced, and could have been triggered by the residual effects of the anesthesia and the pain medication. Dr. R's coming to the hospital made Anna feel that she was not abandoned. She seemed more relaxed the next day when Dr. R called on her again. The dreams had not recurred, and she was discharged from the hospital a couple of days later. Anna continued to see Dr. R for psychotherapy for several months thereafter. At first she was quite distressed about her condition, but gradually, as the pain and discomfort decreased, she began to focus on her work and the pleasurable aspects of her life.

4.3. BREAST CANCER

The results of studies on the emotional adjustment of breast cancer patients are mixed, with some revealing exceptionally good adjustment and others moderate to severe problems. When psychological problems do arise, they seem to peak during the first year after a mastectomy, with a noticeable reduction in stress after two years (Maguire et al., 1978). Should the disease recur, patients may feel even more devastated than the first time. Maguire and her colleagues found that mastectomy patients had a higher incidence of psychiatric complications than did a control group composed of women with benign breast disease. Most of the women with psychological symptoms did not seek help, and of those who did, most received only prescriptions for antianxiety drugs from their primary physicians. Referrals for psychological support were apparently not high on the physicians' agenda, with many assuming that the distress is natural and that eventually patients will come to terms with their condition. Underlying this reluctance to refer patients for psychological help may be the physicians' need to remain in control of the case.

However, Levine et al. (1978) reported that when referrals were made, patients with breast cancer were referred for psychological consultation more often than patients with other types of cancer. It is not clear if this reflects greater emotional disturbance on the part of these patients, or if those making the referrals (mostly male physicians) are reacting to their own feelings about breast cancer and mastectomies. Another possible explanation is related to the interaction of two factors: Women are more likely to show their feelings, and the majority of women affected with cancer have breast cancer. Thus, physicians may be responding to the patients' outward display of emotion.

Those suffering psychological distress may exhibit depression, anxiety, and an impaired self-image (Maguire, Tait, Brooke, Thomas, & Sellwood, 1980). At first there is the fear of dying, then concerns about treatment and its side effects. Eventually, social and personal issues come to the fore more strongly. The women may feel ugly and socially unacceptable, and their sex life may be adversely affected (Maguire *et al.*, 1978).

4.3.1. Incidence

Breast cancer is the leading cause of cancer death in women, second only to lung cancer (American Cancer Society, 1986). About 1 out of 11 women is expected to develop breast cancer during her lifetime. If the tumor is localized, the five-year survival rate is 91%, if it has spread, the rate drops to 59%. Those at greatest risk are women over age 50 with a personal or family history of breast cancer. Other risk factors include never having had children, or having them after the age of 30. This does not bode well for the incidence of breast cancer in the future, given the growing trend for women to delay having children until they have their careers established.

4.3.2. Treatment

The least invasive surgical procedure is a lumpectomy, where only the tumor and a small amount of surrounding tissue are removed. Some lymph nodes may be taken out for examination to see if the disease has spread. In a simple mastectomy, only the breast is removed, and in a modified radical mastectomy, underlying tissue and some lymph nodes in the armpit are removed as well. A radical mastectomy involves removing the breast, auxiliary lymph nodes, and the pectoral muscles. The extent of the surgery affects the amount of residual weakness and disfigurement the woman will experience afterward.

Additional treatment can include hormonal therapy, where drugs are used to prevent growth of hormone-dependent tumor; chemotherapy to destroy cancer cells throughout the system; and radiation therapy to kill cancer cells in the area from which the tumor was removed. This may be in the form of an external beam (X ray) or the implantation of a radioactive isotope for a few days. During the later procedure the patient is "radioactive," and contact with others is restricted. The isolation and feelings of contamination are hard for some patients to endure.

A lumpectomy is preferred by many women who do not want to lose their breast. There may be some disappointment and depression following this operation if patients are unprepared for the subsequent discomfort from the incisions and radiation, which may last for several months. And initially, the breast may not look aesthetic, owing to redness of the skin, hardness of the breast tissue, and itchiness. Oozing infections may also need to be dealt with. Eventually, as these symptoms disappear, patients begin to feel pleased with their choice. However, recurrences can happen. In Anna's case, the cancer had spread to her lymph nodes, and although she had been given chemotherapy as well as radiation therapy, it did not prevent the tumor from recurring.

Case 5

The Altered Face
(Facial Disfigurement)

5.1. ESTHER

Esther was an attractive older woman, of "uncertain age." She arrived at the therapist's office with a large bandage covering half her face. The therapist had been informed by the referring physician, Dr. M, that the patient had had an advanced case of skin cancer (squamous cell carcinoma) that necessitated radical surgery. The resulting wound was very deep, going as far as the bone, and although not visible because of the bandage, half her nose and cheek had been removed. Dr. M wanted Esther to wait a year before beginning reconstructive surgery, to make sure there was no recurrence of disease. In the meantime, Esther would need to take care of the unsightly gaping wound during its healing process.

To prepare himself for working with this patient, the therapist, Dr. P, a psychologist, needed to understand more of what was involved. In doing so, he had to deal with his own reactions to what certainly would not be a pleasant sight. Dr. M offered to show the therapist slides of the wound, which helped prepare him intellectually and emotionally for what was to come.

5.1.1. The Course of Therapy

Diseases or accidents that affect the face are particularly devastating for those, such as Esther, who have narcissistic personalities. However, the course of her adjustment was not atypical for someone with severe facial cancer. At first, Esther worried about death from the disease. As she faced the reality of a series of operations, she worried about dying from the anesthesia. She also worried about possible pain and how successful the plastic surgery would be. And she feared the recurrence of the disease.

During the long period of treatment, she wondered how she would manage socially and occupationally with a bandage on her face, and also with the periodic surgeries cutting into her life. As time went on, and the surgeries appeared to be having some degree of success, she began looking toward the future. Issues revolving around the self-concept emerged, as did nagging questions: "How disfigured will I be?" "Who will I be (now that I am no longer as beautiful or handsome as I once was)?"

Patients who reach the stage of acceptance are usually happy to be alive and accept the less-than perfect result. However, in certain cases, if the patients are emotionally unstable or are left with very debilitating or disfiguring results, they may suffer serious emotional reactions. This fortunately was not the case with Esther.

5.1.1.1. Dealing with Medical Issues

Following the surgery for removal of the tumor, Esther had been too frightened to look at the surgical wound, and thus, she could not perform the required daily cleansing and changing of bandages. For several weeks she had to be assisted by visiting nurses who came to her home. Although she was perfectly well in other ways, her days now revolved around the schedules of the nurses, upon whom she had become dependent, both emotionally and practically. She was terrified about her face, yet as she began to regain her strength, she started resenting her lack of independence.

Dr. M had given Esther an appointment several months hence. His goal was to remove the bandage and have Esther look at the wound for the first time in his presence. Esther had been using therapy to prepare himself for this day. Dr. P, the psychologist, sensing that the patient was emotionally fragile, decided to be with her when the "unveiling" occurred. Dr. M too was relieved to have the added support, since the patient had been somewhat difficult to manage, becoming demonstrably emotional during examinations.

The day arrived. Dr. M removed the bandage. Esther scrutinized the therapist's face, watching for any sign of revulsion or fear. Because of the previous preparation, the therapist was able to look at the wound clinically, controlling his own facial movements, and at Esther's request described objectively what he saw: a deep hole, redness, some bone. When the mirror was finally given to the patient, Esther's only response was "Disgusting!" There was none of the expected hysterics that had dominated her earlier dealings with her illness. She had used the mirroring face of her therapist and the therapist's behavior to prepare herself for what was to come. And as she said later, "It was not as bad as I had built it up to be in my mind."

5.1.1.2. Therapist's Notes

Both of Esther's parents had died of cancer in their 50s, as had her older sister and favorite aunt. Memories of their illnesses and eventual deaths overwhelmed her as she relived these events. Compounding this was Esther's own past history with cancer, having had two mastectomies during the past 10 years. These she had dealt with through denial, and her own fears and narcissistic feelings had not let her work them through. Also, unresolved guilt about her husband's emotional illness and eventual death plagued her now that she too was ill. Excerpts from the therapist's notes reveal how various issues surfaced and resurfaced throughout her extended therapy.

1984

[Following removal of the tumor, but before reconstructive surgery.]

11/2/84. Patient reports that her husband had been treated with electroshock therapy for his depressions. At the time, patient felt that she too was being electrocuted and would shake. Eventually she left her husband, and he died of an aneurysm a few months later. Now she feels that her husband is punishing her for having deserted him, by her having his symptoms, i.e., the shaking. (Doctor's offices and hospitals reminded patient of her husband's treatments. And when she was first diagnosed as having facial cancer, she trembled and cried each time the physician came near her, shaking uncontrollably. Perhaps the bowel problems, of which she also complains, have a psychological basis as well, as her husband also had a colostomy.)

1985

2/27/85. Would like to have sex again, to feel alive before she dies.

3/13/85. Has appointment with surgeon. Is very anxious, trembling, afraid of being disfigured.

Said aunt in her eighties, father's sister, has just been diagnosed with liver cancer. This aunt is the last of that generation. Now Esther is the oldest of her generation, and she too has cancer.

4/2/85. Patient saw Dr. M. Told her she was disease-free. Said her reaction surprised her as she hadn't realized that she was concerned about the disease. Went out and bought herself a robe and new slippers. Starting thinking of the future. Now concerned about cosmetic surgery. Will she look grotesque?

4/30/85. Aunt died. Scattered in sessions, death of aunt, worried about self. Having bowel problems again. Worried about cancer. Anxious. "Who am I?" she asks. "I don't know myself."

5/7/85. Saw surgeon. Reconstructive surgery scheduled for 9/9. Then got confused about the date. Worried about the operation. Scattered throughout sessions. Difficulty staying on one subject. Reflects back to former therapist. He would know what to do. He was like a parent. Not sure if that is what she wants. Wants to be a person. To keep living. Worried about how will get through next four months before the operation. Feels out of control, a victim. Identifies with the holocaust victims. Worried about being able to pay for all the operations.

5/14/85. Saw a man in the lobby of the office building with a large growth on his face. Doesn't want people to see her. Says needs to talk about upcoming operation, but then talks about her children and family problems.

Patient upset as she feels she should be talking about operation, yet doesn't stay on the subject. Keeps talking about wanting to get a puppy, her career and possible additional training, going on a vacation. Told is not getting off the subject, but is talking about some very strong needs: To be loved and loving (complains about her children not being close enough); to get back into life after the operation, to have a future; and the need to be happy. Must remember that she is still a person with a life. Working on these other issues is a way of giving herself strength and hope, and preparing herself for the operation.

9/6/85. Why does she cry when doctors come near her? Because it makes it all real, what she has to go through. Because up to then she could block it out. Denial is the only way to cope. Is like she has a wall around her and they step through, break through the defense. She falls apart, and becomes emotional.

10/1/85. [This session follows the first in a series of operations for reconstructive surgery.] Is going to the surgeon later in the day. Is afraid he will want her to look at her face. Can only look at it a little bit at a time. Doesn't like anyone touching it. Asked me [therapist] to look at it. I [therapist] say is smaller than before. Looks like there is a lot of swelling. Spoke very clinically, but honestly.

10/8/85. Esther looked at her face last week. Said previous session helped to prepare her. Again used therapist as reflecting mirror. Feels it looks like a giant wart. Doesn't like the bloody look. Would eventually like a face lift, to look young.

Esther embarrassed to ask surgeon how long she should wait to use cosmetics and have her hair colored. She was afraid he would consider her questions frivolous. Esther has narcissistic tendencies, and her beauty has always been her entree, both socially and in work. She has often felt like a shell, with beauty as her only asset. Being ill has played havoc with her self-concept and has made her feel older. Esther encouraged to raise the issue of cosmetics and hair coloring with her physician.

10/15/85. Esther pleased that physician treated her vanity concerns seriously, and to her surprise put no restrictions on her use of cosmetics or hair coloring, as the incisions have been healing nicely. Her beautician still is very concerned about working on her, and is trying to talk her out of the hair treatment.

10/22/85. Now that her face is altered she is not sure of her identity. Also she thinks that under the bandage she looks grotesque.

1986

2/18/86. [Has had more surgery, another operation coming up.] Esther is very anxious and scattered. She wants to live, and is afraid she won't make it through next week's surgery. She is also afraid results won't be good, and is coming to the end of the series of operations. Also the surgeon is performing another operation in the morning, and Esther is afraid he will be tired when he gets to her.

6/10/86. Found out that she needs at least two more operations for her reconstructive surgery. Is a set-back that the July operation is not the last. Says not sure could have handled this if knew would need so many. Is using her work to distract her and to pull herself into life.

Also has been advised to get a colonoscopy, and needs two new prostheses re her mastectomy. She has also discovered a small lump on her leg.

8/12/86. Rather than denial is now becoming hypervigilant. Esther feels there is a growth that is getting bigger on other side of her face. Says it is different from previous one.

[Countertransference reaction: Dr. P finds himself feeling down, as he has worked with this patient for several years helping her get through all the operations, and helping her to deal with the pain and possibility of deformity. Now that the end is almost in sight, another tumor may be raising its ugly head. Just isn't fair, and is frightening.]

Patient read a pamphlet by a psychologist who had had the same operation. She said she could not read it when it was first given to her, as was too threatening.

Tries to stick to the notes that she brings with her. Too painful to let her thoughts roam. When gets off her notes talks about her mastectomy. Doesn't want anyone to know. Feels will be looked down upon. Can't get too close to anyone. Feels men won't want her because of her mastectomy, and now her face just makes it more impossible. She doesn't like to shop for clothes. Limits her life. Says misses her breasts, liked them.

[Note. Esther has refused to look at her body in a mirror, since her mastectomies ten years ago. At the time, she withdrew physically from her husband, never speaking of her reasons, not even facing them herself. Now a widow for the past six years, she is beginning to realize that her avoidance of having a relationship with a man, and her rejection of her body have come about from her excessive use of denial. Although this defense had served her well during the initial stages of her illness, and even helped her get through other very difficult times, it had eventually limited her personal growth and interpersonal interactions.]

Is getting her apartment redone, cleaning, ironing her clothes. Preparing for the fall operation in an orderly way. (Is she preparing for death or for the future?)

9/30/86. Surgeon took off three more lesions from her leg, all benign. Patient shook like a child. Feels like he is a grandfather to her. The burning of her skin to remove the lesions reminded her of her grandmother's singeing chickens.

Saw a man in the waiting room with no hands. Feels like they are taking pieces of her body, bit by bit.

Plastic surgeon explained that the reason she has been so upset is that she had to walk around with a hole in her face for a year. Esther said she hadn't thought of that. Had treated it as if were not a part of her body. It was the only way she could survive what she had to go through.

Esther is upset about her appearance. She feels she is going to be disfigured by her lip, which now droops slightly. Surgeon explained that in a museum you look at the whole. If you tear it apart, will see flaws here and there, but when you consider the entire work, the flaws are not noticeable. Patient was relieved somewhat by his poetic explanation.

1988

[This patient is still in psychotherapy, and facing the last of the reconstructive surgeries. Although the results are not as perfect as she had hoped, they are remarkable, and she gets compliments on her appearance from strangers as well as friends. She is working full time in a new position that brings her into constant contact with the public every day, and she is getting about more easily socially. However, she is now faced with personal and interpersonal problems that she had been able to avoid when she had the facial disfigurement and the operations to use as an excuse.]

5.2. FACIAL DISFIGUREMENT

The face more than any other part of the body represents one's identity. It is what you present to the world. Others recognize you by your face, and react to you in terms of its appearance. Its imperfections are not easily hidden, and people considered ugly, repulsive, or distorted may become the object of discrimination or ridicule.

A facial deformity can result from a wide variety of circumstances, such as an automobile accident, an explosion or fire, a physical assault such as a knifing, a disease, or a congenital abnormality. Surgery or radiation therapy may be required to save the person's life or help him or her regain function. But these same beneficial treatments can leave their own deforming marks, emotionally and physically. Patients may need to be subjected to a series of operations over a period of years, each time having to deal with the mounting anxiety over the fear of pain, and the uncertainty of how successful the surgery will be. And in the end there may nevertheless be residual scarring, or muscle or nerve damage.

New advances in plastic surgery and other restorative techniques can produce results that appear miraculous in many cases, when one considers the extent of the original disease or trauma (Hoban, 1984). However, the psychological consequences of having had a disfigured face may continue long after reconstructive surgery has been performed. And the emotional distress is not necessarily in proportion to the severity of the original disfigurement, or to the actual outcome of the surgery (Macgregor, 1984). The ability to accept the new and altered face is related to the person's fantasies and expectations, the patient's psychological makeup, and the reactions from others throughout the ordeal.

5.2.1. Facial Cancer

Skin cancer is one possible cause of facial deformity. Although the current popular thought is that skin cancer is not serious and can be cured, it is not always that simple, particularly for the more advanced or aggressive tumors. Facial cancers usually can be treated, however, if caught early. Unfortunately, there is the tendency for people to delay going for treatment, either minimizing the threat or fearing the diagnosis, which brings up associations of death, social rejection, pain, and suffering (Freidenbergs, 1981).

If treatment is delayed, however, the skin tumor may spread or invade deep into the tissue, which could necessitate the removal of large sections of the face, part of the nose, or possibly an eye or an ear. And some skin cancers can metastasize to other parts of the body, or recur again on the face, if all the cancerous tissue has not been excised. And some tumors, if not caught early or properly treated, can result in death.

Although plastic surgery techniques today are so advanced that they can achieve what formerly would have been considered miraculous reconstructions, the results do not always restore the person's function and looks to what they once were (Goldwyn, 1984). When cancer strikes the head or neck, it brings with it the added problems that communication, eating, and breathing may be impaired (Harris, Vogtsberger, & Mattox, 1985). Nerve and muscle damage may interfere with expression, sensation, and speaking. Smiles may be distorted, and there may be drooling. The person's nose may run without his being aware of it, or the mouth may droop. Patients may feel that they look grotesque and repulsive, as they notice the quickly averted glances or stares of others (Turns & Sands, 1978). Both men and women can find their self-concept shattered, and their lives restricted socially and occupationally (Turkington, 1984).

Case 6

The Devil Inside (Seizure Disorder)

When Pat entered the room for her first session, she looked quite cheery. She had just come from working out at the health club, where she also worked part time while going to graduate school. Pat had been referred for psychotherapy by a physician in whom she had confided. Underneath the bubbly facade was a frightened, depressed, and angry 25-year-old.

Pat originally began having petit mal seizures when she was 15, following a case of meningitis. For a long time the seizures did not interfere with her functioning and were totally controlled by drugs. The month she was to graduate from college, her doctor had decided to take her off the medication. He had been having her taper down on the dosage, but unbeknownst to him Pat had decided that she wanted to be totally drug-free by graduation day. She speeded up the process. A week before graduation she had her first grand mal seizure.

Now in graduate school, Pat was having difficulty concentrating. She would have blackouts, causing her to forget what she had just read, or what the professor had said before. Pat was not as far along in her education as she would have liked because of the disruptions caused by her illness.

Years before, her neurologist had suggested surgery as a possibility. She had put it off; it seemed so frightening. But the pattern of seizures kept repeating itself. Pat would be placed on a new drug regime, and for the first three or four weeks she would be seizure-free. Then gradually the blackouts and petit mals would recur, and sometimes grand mals.

Pat was at her wits' end; she felt she could not go on. Finally she agreed to the operation. The very idea terrified her: that they would put her to sleep, that they would cut open her head and go probing around in her brain. Maybe they would make a mistake.

In the months before surgery, Pat began acting out, exhibiting self-denigrating and self-destructive behavior. She began drinking heavily, which was against her doctor's orders, and started picking up strangers in bars for "one-night stands." "I thought I was going to die, so why not" was the way she explained it later. "And I was mad at God." Deep inside she felt she was not a worthy person, and she was punishing herself. Later, she would feel guilty about her behavior.

In the first therapy session, Pat's initial high spiritedness cracked, exposing her despair. Apparently the operation had not been as successful as she had hoped. They were not able to remove all of the lesion. During the first month following the surgery she was seizure-free, but gradually she began having the blackouts and petit mals. At the time she began therapy, she was having at least three blackouts a day, and about five petit mals a week. "They promised me everything would be OK," she would repeat woefully, again and again.

The referring physician had described Pat as a determined young woman. She wanted to do all those things that people said she would not be able to do, and to do them well. She had always been athletic as a little girl, and felt that her body cried out for movement. Despite the possibility of seizures, she jogged, she did aerobics, she used Nautilus machines, and she played on a women's softball team on Saturdays. Sometimes she blacked out during these activities, but over time, as those around her began to understand her condition, they would patiently wait for her to regain consciousness and would help her as needed.

Pat reported being upset about the lack of control in front of others. She said she particularly didn't want strangers to know what was wrong. Even though she didn't want them to know, she would become upset if they thought she was drunk. She also feared hurting herself during a seizure, particularly her eyes. So far, except for some minor bruises, outwardly there were no major scars.

Pat was upset when she came to her second therapy session. She had had a petit mal while teaching aerobics. She was concerned that she might have to give up her job at the health club. She had also had two seizures the night before, and in anger had torn off her medical ID bracelet, identifying her as an epileptic, a label she had resisted for a long time.

Pat blamed the blackouts on the Dilantin level's being too high, and said that it was being adjusted by her new physician. She had decided to see a different neurologist, since the one she had been going to had ruled out strenuous sports. Pat could not accept this and claimed she needed the activity to burn off tension. Perhaps the new doctor would agree with her. Although she was willing to talk in therapy about alternatives to her strenuous exercises, it seemed to be mostly to please the therapist, who was also concerned about her stressful activities. Pat was determined not to let the disorder stop her. On the surface the determination was admirable, but psychological denial was strong, possibly to the point of being self-destructive.

Pat did not keep her next two appointments. Attempts to reach her were futile. Then she called and came in for an appointment. She was very despondent. Her appointment with the new neurologist had been very upsetting. Not only had he not supported her continuing to do strenuous exercise, he also mentioned the possibility of further surgery—and this time with no guarantees. Pat said the last surgery had been the worst time of her life. She saw the new neurologist as cold and insensitive, and felt he didn't understand how upsetting the idea of a second operation was to her.

At the end of the session Pat admitted that she had been feeling suicidal after her visit to the doctor. She had a lot of medication in her apartment, where she lived alone, and was afraid that sometime she might take it when she is feeling down. Pat said that she did not want to die, that she was determined to live, but felt overwhelmed by it all. The therapist suggested that she leave her medicine with her neighbor, who was also a close friend, and keep on hand only the minimum necessary. Pat accepted this idea readily, and in fact seemed relieved by it. As she was leaving the session, she mentioned that she was going to call her neighbor as soon as she got home.

At the next session Pat confided that she had been feeling depressed and suicidal the previous evening. She said that she had called a couple of friends and they had come to stay with her. She said that she was glad she had moved her medication to her neighbor's place, that it made her feel more secure.

She also confided to the therapist for the first time that she had actually tried to kill herself about a year before. She had "blacked out" and upon waking up found herself quite far from home. She could hear some young men taunting her about being drunk. She said she was angry and humiliated, but could not react. She wanted to yell at them but couldn't speak. A woman came up to her and, noticing her medical ID bracelet, asked if she were OK. By then, Pat had regained all her senses but felt very tired. She was pleased when the woman offered to escort her home. She assured the samaritan that she was all right, but as the evening wore on and she was alone, she kept thinking of those fellows calling her names and teasing her. In anger, she impulsively grabbed a bottle of aspirin and swallowed all the pills that were in it. She couldn't remember how many there were. She fell asleep and was sick for three days. This was a serious attempt, since she had even written notes to her parents and her best friend from childhood.

Pat reiterated that she really didn't want to die, that she believed these deep depressions were from the medication. She said she had been on tranquilizers when she had made the suicide attempt, and felt they were responsible. She again expressed anger at the new physician and said that he had put her on a different drug and she felt he hadn't listened when she said she couldn't take tranquilizers.

Eventually, the levels of the medication seemed to be corrected again, and Pat was seizure-free for several weeks. During this time she gained some perspective on her reactions to those treating her, particularly her physicians, who took the brunt of her anger. But Pat lashed out in all directions. She was fighting with some of her friends and with her parents. Although she had told the therapist earlier that she could not have made it without her, she tended to miss sessions when things were not going well and when she was angry.

Pat expressed her upset at "feeling like an outsider." "I want to be treated like others," she explained, "not excluded." She said that when she has a seizure people pull away. Then, afterward, when she is depressed or wants to talk about it, she has been accused of self-pity. She explained that some of her friends react this way when they are trying to encourage her to be strong, but that it is the wrong thing to do. Sympathizing, saying, "You must be depressed," or asking, "Do you want to talk or be left alone?" feels better. Pat said that having epilepsy makes you feel lower than others, that you have to show them, that you have to be better and do more than what they say you can do. If people (i.e., her parents) tell her that she shouldn't do something, then she does. Just to show them. She wants to be free.

At the therapist's suggestion, Pat attended a group meeting of persons with seizure disorders. Many were much older than she and were working in a variety of jobs. Pat found the meeting quite encouraging and was thinking that maybe she too could adjust to having the seizures. When the academic year ended, Pat returned to her family home for the summer. She said that she would get in touch with the therapist in the fall, but did not. The therapist learned from the referring physician that Pat was still quite depressed and was considering a second operation, with no guarantees.

6.2. Seizure Disorder

Epilepsy is a neurological condition characterized by a variety of symptoms, such as muscle spasms, mental confusion, loss of consciousness, and uncontrolled or aimless body movements. These changes are referred to as epileptic seizures, and the condition itself is frequently called a seizure disorder. The condition is not a single unitary disorder but a complexity of clinical phenomena. Although the seizures can range from mild to severe, they usually last only a short while. There may be as many as 20 a day, or as few as 1 every year or so. Although most persons with seizure disorders lead normal, unrestricted lives, about 15 to 20% are significantly restricted by their seizures (Kaplan & Wyler, 1983).

That the brain is the center of this disorder was not confirmed until the advent of the electroencephalogram (EEG) in 1929. Although much still remains to be understood, the general thesis is that epilepsy results from brief, abnormal electrical discharges in the brain. During a seizure, an unusual amount of electrical energy passes between cells, either overloading a specific area or swamping the brain's whole system (Epilepsy Foundation of

America, 1982, 1983). There are many possible causes of this abnormality: birth defects, head injuries, diseases such as measles or encephalitis, disorders of the circulatory system, tumors. In many cases the cause is not known.

Grand mal or generalized tonic-clonic seizures result in the convulsive movements often associated in the public's eye with epilepsy. These may start with a sudden cry, caused by air being suddenly forced out of the lungs. The person falls to the ground unconscious; the body stiffens briefly, then there are sudden jerking movements. Bladder or bowel control is sometimes lost. A frothy saliva may appear around the mouth. Shallow breathing or temporarily suspended breathing may occur, and the skin may turn bluish. The movements then gradually slow down as the seizure ends normally, all this usually occurring in no more than two to five minutes.

After regaining consciousness, the person may be confused or tired, having no memory of what has happened. He or she may experience a headache or have difficulty speaking. Rest or sleep may be needed. In most cases, after resting for a while, the person can resume normal activities. This type of seizure may be mistaken for a heart attack or a stroke.

Petit mal or absence seizures are nonconvulsive seizures that may take the form of "blanking out," including brief staring spells, slight twitching, rapid blinking, chewing movements, and loss of awareness. Observers may mistake these seizures for daydreaming or deliberate lack of attention.

Psychomotor or temporal lobe seizures usually start with a blank stare, followed by chewing movements, and then random activity. Sufferers may seem dazed and unaware of their surroundings. They may mumble, and their actions may be clumsy and not directed. They may run or appear afraid, yet struggle if someone tries to restrain them. Although this behavior may last for only a few minutes, the confusion afterward can be substantially longer, and there is no memory of what has happened. It is not hard to imagine that those witnessing such behavior might mistake it for drunkenness, drug abuse, or mental illness. Half of all those with epilepsy suffer from temporal lobe seizures, and more than half of those also suffer generalized, grand mal seizures.

Myoclonic seizures are sudden brief, massive muscle jerks that may involve the whole body or a part of the body, such as an arm or a leg. This behavior may cause such persons to spill what they are holding or to fall off the chair. In a public place this may be mistaken for clumsiness or bizarre behavior.

6.2.1. What to Do

Should a patient have a convulsive seizure, try to stay calm. Do not try to restrain him. If he is seated when the seizure starts, ease him to the floor if possible. Remove hazards such as hard or sharp objects that could cause injury if the person were to fall or knock against them. Loosen tight clothing and, if he is wearing glasses, remove them. Help protect his airways by gently turning him on his side so that any fluid in the mouth can drain safely. Never try to force the mouth open. Let the seizure run its course. When it ends, let the person rest. Be calm and reassuring, since the patient may feel embarrassed or disoriented.

If you know the patient is prone to seizures, there is no need to call an ambulance if (1) the seizure ends in under 10 minutes, (2) consciousness returns without further incident, and (3) there are no signs of injury or other serious problems. If there is no known history and the patient is not wearing a medical ID bracelet or necklace, then you should call an ambulance if the seizure continues for more than 5 minutes. This precaution is recommended in case the seizure is caused by another condition (Epilepsy Foundation of America, 1983).

Should a patient experience a nonconvulsive seizure, speak calmly and reassuringly, and if necessary gently guide the patient away from obvious hazards. Don't grab her, because she may struggle or lash out at you. Stay with her until she is completely aware of where she is, and offer to help get her home. If you are not able to accompany her yourself because of other appointments, do your best to find someone else who can.

6.2.2. Medical Treatment

Seizure control is attempted through the use of anticonvulsive and antiepileptic drugs, the most common of which are Dilantin, Phenobarbital, Zarontin, Tegretol, and Tranzene. Valium may also be used. These drugs do not cure the condition, but in 50% of the cases the seizures can be completely controlled, and reduced in another 30 to 35%. Unfortunately for some people, the dosage may need to be adjusted every three months or so (Gilman, Goodman, & Gilman, 1980). A recurrence of seizures can be very depressing for a patient who has been almost seizure-free and now feels that treatment has not worked.

Surgery may be used in selected cases when medication has not been effective, and the seizures severely encumber the person's life. Surgery is tried only when it is determined that the lesion is in a single small part of the brain that can be removed safely without damaging brain function or personality. The surgery is apparently safe, since fewer than 1% die as a result of the operation. However, the prognosis is uncertain. Results of surgical excision are typically as follows: 30% become seizure-free, 50% have significant reduction in the number of seizures (i.e., greater than 60% reduction), and for 20% there is no effect (Kaplan & Wyler, 1983, p. 265). For this group the disappointment is tremendous, since surgery is often seen as the last hope, and patients undertake it with great expectations, despite all the cautions and qualifications they have heard.

6.2.3. Interpersonal Issues and Mental Health

A social stigma has hung over epilepsy for centuries. Pictures of uncontrolled flailing and thrashing of limbs horrified the uneducated public, who thought the person was possessed by the devil. In some societies, persons with epilepsy were treated as untouchables or mentally ill. Other societies, however, relegated them to the position of mystics with special powers (Kaplan & Wyler, 1983).

Although about 1 person in 100 has epilepsy, in many cases friends and associates may not be aware of it. Between episodes the person will be quite normal, except for possible psychological problems that may arise from the person's own feelings and the reactions of others to the seizures.

Counseling and psychotherapy have been recommended as an adjunct to medical care (Max, 1980). Fear of rejection may lead to secrecy that imposes feelings of guilt, shame, fears of punishment, and denigration of the sense of self. Living with the fear of ostracism, with the feeling that somehow you are less than others, plagues many people with seizure disorders. They may also fear not being able to live normal lives, i.e., to get married and have children, or to work at a profession or job of their choice. Although only 15 to 20% of those with seizure disorders have lives that are significantly restricted by their seizures, the underlying fears remain for many. In some cases the condition may lead to fear of intimacy: The person may shun interpersonal relationships or, on the contrary, have many superficial ones.

One infuriating problem is that certain seizures may be mistaken for drunkenness or being high on drugs. Patients may stagger, walk clumsily, bump into people and objects. The person may awake to hear comments such as "You should be ashamed of yourself, being drunk in the middle of the day." Anger and shame can cause a frustrating rage. Patients have been known to withdraw and become severely depressed after such incidents. An individual may dread the possibility of an attack occurring in public, even after many years of having the seizures under control. Some may become socially withdrawn and hesitant to try new things.

Children with epilepsy are likely to experience overprotectiveness and overindulgence, resulting in later adjustment problems (Zeigler, 1981). Such parental reactions are particularly difficult for the adolescent with a seizure disorder who is trying to deal with issues of independence and separation. Acting-out behavior can take the form of excessive use of alcohol and illegal drugs, sexual acting-out, or "overdoing" in activities (e.g., trying to show that they are as good as or better than others—for instance, by excelling in sports). Although moderate exercise is thought to be good for seizure control (possibly because of tension reduction), patients trying to prove themselves may overdo in this area, putting excess strain on the system.

People with temporal lobe epilepsy are thought by some to be emotionally labile and prone to violent behavior (Bear & Fedio, 1977; Hermann &

Chhabria, 1980). Also, psychoticlike behavior has been observed following the surgical removal of a temporal lobe for psychomotor epilepsy.

When personality, emotional, and behavioral changes do occur, any of a host of symptoms may present themselves: heightened emotional intensity, rapid mood changes, paranoid episodes, hallucinations and delusions, hysterical symptoms, anxiety, depersonalization (feeling oneself or one's body to be unreal), drug and alcohol abuse, sleep and appetite changes, and loss of sexual interest and capacity. Although the psychological symptoms may be controlled by anticonvulsant drugs, the drugs themselves may cause dulling, depression, and behavioral changes (Blumer, 1986). In fact, the symptoms of epilepsy present themselves like many psychiatric illnesses and are often misdiagnosed.

The extent of psychological complications, however, has been questioned, and the issue of psychosis and epilepsy is controversial (Hermann, Schwartz, Whitman, & Karnes, 1980; Pritchard, Lombroso, & McIntyre, 1980; Stevens, 1975, 1980; D.C. Taylor, 1975). Blumer (1986) feels that the psychiatric aspects of epilepsy have been neglected in recent years, as professionals attempt to combat the social prejudices that have existed over the centuries. He points out that the temporal-limbic system plays an important role in regulating emotions and behavior. Thus, one might expect some personality changes if that area of the nervous system is affected by the epilepsy. In fact, he states that psychiatric disorders may result without evidence of the seizures typically associated with temporal lobe epilepsy. Proper diagnosis is important so that proper medication can be given. It should be emphasized that these symptoms are experienced by a minority of epileptic patients, but therapists need to be aware of the possible relationship between an epileptic disorder and such symptoms.

Case 7

Like a Leper (Venereal Disease)

7.1. THE GROUP

The case studies that follow are based on several members of a genital herpes group, and illustrate the interaction of the psychological, social, and ethical issues associated with having a venereal disease. Psychological factors, including stress, depression, anxiety, and interpersonal problems, are thought to influence the course of genital herpes infections (Levenson, Hamer, Meyers, Hart, & Kaplowitz, 1987). To help patients deal with these psychological issues, the group therapy made use of a combination of psychodynamic and cognitive–behavioral techniques. Sessions would start with imagery and relaxation exercises to help the patients relax and learn how to handle bodily stress, and then would move on to either assertiveness training, sharing of experiences, sharing of information, or role playing.

Assertiveness training was approached at first in a general way, i.e., helping the patients to become more direct in their life situations. It was felt that if they did not incorporate the principles of assertiveness in their overall functioning, they would have difficulty doing so in relation to their stressful illness. One of the main areas where the patients had difficulty being assertive was in telling a potential sexual partner that they had a herpes infection. Role playing was one of the techniques used to develop the skills needed and to examine the related feelings.

7.1.1. Jean

Jean, a 32-year-old schoolteacher, had a herpes infection for at least 10 years before joining the group. She did not think much about it until it became one of the media's sensational topics. When she joined the group she was very worried. She thought about her body almost all the time in an obsessive way, feeling unclean and contagious, like a leper. She effectively had no social life to speak of, neither with women nor with men. She had never felt attractive, and having herpes just added to her poor self-image.

Jean had a stocky build. She was what would be described as plain, wearing no makeup, and her very oily hair was worn quite short. At times she reported having bulimic tendencies, and her appearance could change dramatically, depending upon her mood and related eating habits. When she was feeling down or anxious, she would binge on junk food, reportedly putting on many pounds in a few hours. She insightfully described this as part of her self-destructiveness.

Her self-pity was enormous, and she often portrayed herself as someone who was so badly off that she just couldn't be helped. When help was offered, she would respond by saying, "You couldn't possibly understand anyway." During her absence at one session, the group members talked of their hesitancies about confronting her. They felt that Jean had a very aggressive and angry way of responding when suggestions or criticisms were offered, and that she used her illnesses, i.e., the herpes and bulimia, as diversions to keep from dealing with other personal issues.

Jean often acted as the "interviewer," or tried to play the role of therapist in the group, directing a series of questions to one person and at times cutting other group members out of the interaction. Part of this great interest in others was a way of staying in control and avoiding revealing her own feelings. Her participation in the role playing was at first as teacher, the one who would show the others how they might behave or feel. Later, however, she began to let go of her defensiveness and let herself participate in the interactions.

Jean could not explain how she might have contracted herpes. Her sexual experiences were very limited, and she was vague when pressed for details about them. The only emotional involvement she had had in recent years was with Paul, a homosexual man who had not been sexually active since the AIDS epidemic became known. Jean said they had never had intercourse but were physically close, kissing and petting. He lived far away but came to town three or four times a year for personal and business reasons. She looked forward to seeing him, and, in fact, her appearance changed quite dramatically when he was around. She would use makeup, style her hair, and don a skirt rather than her usual slacks. It was noted by the group that her mood became more positive as well.

The group raised the question as to whether her having herpes had anything to do with her nonsexual involvement with Paul. She denied this, stating that he was happy with the relationship the way it was. The question was also raised as to her choice of a currently asexual (or homosexual) partner for a long-term relationship, as well as a person who was not available much of the year.

After several months, Jean began talking about wanting to marry Paul. She expressed uneasiness about what his reaction might be to the herpes, that he might think that she had been promiscuous, or that he might pull away from her for fear of getting the disease himself. The group pointed out that he was already about as far away as he could get, and they encouraged her either to approach him with the subject or to forget him and get on with her life. Although Jean professed wanting a more intimate sexual relationship with a man, she was hesitant to be more assertive with Paul for fear of losing him entirely, and finding someone else to be close to would be difficult for her. When the group terminated, Jean was considering going into individual psychotherapy to work on the underlying conflicts regarding her interpersonal problems and self-image.

7.1.2. Samantha

Samantha, a 20-year-old college junior, had just contracted herpes a few months before joining the group. She had been very popular and said she had often been described as having a "bubbly personality." But since her first outbreak, she had been quite depressed. She had been dating Bob, also a college student, for two years; however, a few months ago, the relationship had begun to sour. Bob had suggested that they start dating other people which Samantha had already been doing for some time without his knowledge.

Depressed and unsure of her own desirability, Samantha began frequenting the local college hangouts. One night she met a 50-year-old lawyer. They had a "one-night stand," and not long thereafter she was diagnosed as having herpes. Samantha berated herself. She hadn't even liked the man. She had no desire to see him again. Why had she not had the courage to say no? Why had she gone to his place? The questions plagued her. Then her anger turned from herself to the man. Why hadn't he told her he had herpes? How could he have done that to her?

Her outbreaks were quite frequent, once a month, and quite virulent. She had been reassured by her physician that they would probably subside as time went on, but for now they were painful and a nuisance, to say the least.

Samantha learned in the group about a doctor who specialized in herpes. She also heard others discuss clever ideas they had discovered to avoid spreading the infection—for example, drying the area with paper towels or a hair dryer after washing. Samantha expressed a feeling of comfort in meeting others who had the condition, and learning how they handled themselves socially. She had previously thought of herself as a sexually attractive, free-spirited person. Now she was confused. What would happen to her? Would she be able to date? Marry? Have children?

She struggled with the ethical issues of if, when, and whom to tell about her herpes. She was shocked to learn that one could not be 100% sure that the infection was not contagious between outbreaks. Some literature said there was a shedding of virus right before and right after an outbreak, but how would she know when this might occur, since she did not have predromal symptoms?

During group, Samantha participated readily in the role playing, trying to learn how she might broach the subject when meeting men she found attractive. Sometimes she played the person with the infection: "There's something I need to discuss with you...." And sometimes she had the chance to play the role of the partner, trying to be understanding or being the one to recoil and be rejecting. The group provided a forum for her to openly discuss her conflicted feelings, and challenged her as she contemplated not telling a new male interest about the herpes, particularly if she were between outbreaks. The group confronted her: Would she be acting out—doing to a man what she felt had been done to her (i.e., not telling, and giving him herpes)?

Samantha struggled with how and when to tell a date, particularly someone she really liked. Would he reject her? Should she get to know him first, let him get to know her, then he'd be less likely to pull away? Or would he then feel angered and betrayed if he hadn't been told earlier? How could she handle it if after being informed, he didn't call her again? Through the weeks of group therapy, Samantha struggled with her conflict, testing out her ideas and feelings in the group. Eventually, she had the opportunity to put some of the role playing into practice, and she shared her experiences with the group.

By termination Samantha reported feeling better about herself, although much less confident than before. She had resumed her relationship with Bob, who had been told about the herpes and had been understanding. She was still tentative about him, having felt betrayed by both him and her 50-year-old one-night stand. However, Bob's willingness to resume a sexual and intimate relationship with her again, knowing of her condition, made her feel less desperate about her situation.

7.1.3. Ray

Ray was a 24-year-old white male homosexual who worked as a waiter. He had few friends and was basically very lonely. Even in the group he felt isolated, being the only male for a time, and the only homosexual.

Ray often felt that his problems were not important and that others weren't interested in them. Thus, for long periods he would remain silent. When this was brought to his attention, he discussed his feeling that people were not interested in him and did not care for him.

Ray had a number of personal problems and crises during the year. His frequent sexual encounters had led to venereal diseases of various sorts, which made him feel unattractive and not clean. He was afraid of getting AIDS but had not always practiced safe sex. He seemed to relish describing his sexual encounters to the women in specific detail. Since gay men were becoming more health-conscious, his outbreaks of herpes had caused several new friends to pull away. Between outbreaks Ray did not tell lovers that he had herpes. He felt that it would further alienate them from him.

Ray envied the women in the group for having found a gynecologist who specialized in herpes, and he wished that he could see their physician. This was not possible, however, since gynecologists, because of their specialty, can treat only women. Ray had been seen by a gay physician; however, that man had contracted AIDS and was no longer in practice. Ray was now alone with his illnesses. He felt that his sexual activity had self-destructive qualities to it, and he saw the herpes as a warning, something that might help him limit his obsessive need for sex with different partners.

In the group Ray initially had difficulty getting involved in the behaviorally oriented exercises. He was very self-conscious and would tend to laugh and make jokes, as a way of distancing himself. But he attended the sessions regularly and did keep up with the reading. As the months passed, he was able to participate more effectively in the assertiveness and role playing.

By the end of therapy, Ray had found himself another physician, one who was sympathetic to his plight and had considerable experience with venereal disease. He seemed to have modified his sexual adventures (although it may have been his reports that were modified with the advent of Jack—a macho professed heterosexual—into the group).

Also, by the end of the year, Ray had decided to move to Provincetown with his ex-wife and ex-lover. He felt that these were his family, since his own family had disowned him many years before. His attempts to cut back on his sexual activity, or at least to be more selective, had reduced the disgust that he had expressed toward his body. Ray obviously had made some progress as a result of the group, but there was certainly much more work to be done. He was encouraged to continue in therapy, either group or individual, once he got settled in his new home.

7.1.4. Jack

Jack, a 33-year-old computer programmer, was unemployed at the time he joined the group. He had been married for 10 years but was now separated from his wife, who threatened to file for divorce. About a year before joining the group, Jack had his first outbreak of herpes. At the time he was not sure what it was, and since it went away he forgot about it. However, when it recurred a few months later, he became concerned and went to a doctor.

Once he learned the diagnosis, he was afraid to tell his wife for fear of her reaction. So he avoided her physically during periods of outbreaks, which lasted about five to six days. A good friend of his had herpes, and the friend's wife never got it, so Jack felt that Ursula was safe.

However, after a few months, Ursula developed a lesion and a month later had a very painful outbreak. Her gynecologist confirmed the diagnosis. Confused and suspicious, Ursula confronted Jack. She had a very volatile personality, so at first Jack denied having herpes himself. But when his next outbreak occurred, it became difficult not to tell her, so he did.

Infuriated that he had been so cruel as not to have told her immediately that he had infected her, she flew into a rage. When pressed as to where he had picked up the virus, Jack again found himself having to lie to her. The truth was that Jack had been having an affair for years with a woman at work. She too was married, and it had never occurred to him that she would provide any risks of this sort. He insisted to his wife that he did not know how he got it—perhaps at the gym. But Ursula was not satisfied.

A narcissistic woman, proud of her beauty and attractiveness, she now felt disgusted with herself and with Jack. She ordered him out of the house. Jack went into a deep depression. He moved in with his mother and in the evenings starting drinking heavily. Eventually he lost his job.

Jack's ego had not been strong even before. He was basically weak and had been very dependent on Ursula. He had used his affair to bolster his ego, yet never had considered leaving his wife. He felt dominated by her, overpowered by her, but prided himself on being an attentive husband. His secrecies had led to the downfall of his marriage, yet the idea of confronting her had been too overwhelming.

In the group Jack first assumed a somewhat macho, arrogant pose. Initially, his hesitancies about being involved were understandable. Joining four months after the group had formed, he was viewed as an outsider. The other members had formed a somewhat cohesive unit. At the same time, his arrival as the second male in a group dominated by females had been anxiously awaited by all.

At first Jack's comments served mostly as a distraction from what was going on. He would move the discussion away from an individual member's personal concerns, taking a more philosophical stance. He would intellectualize and cite statistics whenever possible; when speaking about himself, he tended to refer to a generalized third party, such as "people in their thirties" or "twentieth-century men." This irritated and alienated the other group members, who eventually confronted him on his distant and intellectualizing style.

Jack talked more easily about others' conditions but had great difficulty speaking of his own. His secrecy, which had resulted in the dissolution of his marriage, surfaced in the group. At first he could not discuss openly how he had contracted the infection, at one time implying that his wife might have given it to him.

Eventually, he talked openly about the guilt he felt for what he had done to his wife, both his adulterous affair and the herpes. At times, however, his anger surfaced, bubbling from the conflict over his dependency and her dominance. He hoped subconsciously that she would get herpes: Would it be something they then shared, or something "to bring her down a peg," as he once remarked?

Developmental issues surfaced as Jack spoke of his overpowering mother and his deceased alcoholic father. Jack's poor self-image even before the onset of herpes became evident. In the group Jack eventually was able to understand some of the aspects of his character that had led him to handle his herpes infection in the way he did with his wife. At times he would hide behind his macho stance and attempt to fall back on intellectualization as his defense. He made use of some of the cognitive–behavioral techniques, such as the assertiveness training, which helped him to find a new job and move out on his own again. Opening up discussion with his wife was another matter, since she seemed intent upon getting a divorce. Was she using the herpes as an excuse to end a relationship that had been unsatisfactory for a long time? Or was she angry with Jack for giving her the infection, and for the secrecy and suspected infidelity?

At termination, Jack was learning how to be more open about his vulnerabilities, and he had begun to date. He was still secretive at times when first meeting a woman but at the group's urging had begun trying to be more open about his condition. The fear of rejection was strong. And he was still hoping to get Ursula to reconsider. Jack had a lot more work to do.

7.2. GENITAL HERPES: BACKGROUND

Venereal disease (VD) has plagued mankind since recorded history. In modern times, with the discovery of penicillin and other antibiotics, men and women did not worry about the ravages of VD as they once did. Yet in recent years, the incidence of VD has been on the rise. This increase has been attributed to more persons having multiple sex partners, and the fact that some strains of the infecting agents have become resistant to the antibiotic treatments. Then there are diseases, such as herpes and AIDS, for which no cure has yet been found.

7.2.1. What Is Herpes?

Genital herpes is a viral infection, affecting more than 20 million Americans, with new cases occurring each year. There are two different kinds of herpes simplex. In the past, they could usually be recognized by place of occurrence on the body: HSV-1, or Type 1, appearing above the waist, most commonly around the mouth as a "cold sore" or "fever blister;" and HSV2, or Type 2, appearing below the waist, usually in the genital area. However, as a result of the increase in oral/genital sex, both types have been known to cause lesions in the mouth, as well as in the genital area (Block, 1980; Davis & Keeney, 1981).

Genital herpes causes painful sores which look like blisters or small bumps, and which can rupture to form open sores. In women, the lesions appear inside the vagina, on the cervix, or on the labia; in men, on the penis; and in both sexes, around the anus, thighs, or buttocks. Other accompanying symptoms may be fever, enlarged lymph nodes, and flulike symptoms. The frequency of occurrence can vary from once a month to once a year, or, for some luckier people, only once in a lifetime. But on the average, patients experience about four herpes outbreaks a year (Corey, Adams, Brown, & Holmes, 1983).

The herpes virus enters the skin through mucous membranes and moves along neural pathways into the dorsal root ganglion at the base of the spinal cord. Following the initial, primary infection, the virus lies dormant in the sacral ganglion until there are recurrences, during which time it travels back to the genital area and causes new skin lesions.

Although there is no known cure for herpes, there is symptomatic treatment for the discomfort. Some treatments hasten healing, others are used to prevent infections of the sores. Women who have herpes have an increased risk of cervical cancer, and there are also possible complications during pregnancy (Grossman, Wallen, & Sever, 1981; Nahmias, Naib, & Josey, 1974). If a pregnant woman has active herpes at the time of delivery, the unborn child may get herpes while passing through the vagina during birth. This can result in brain damage to the child or even death. If the mother's herpes infection cannot be effectively treated, a Caesarean section may be necessary to protect the baby's health.

7.2.2. The Personal Dimension

Many people who developed genital herpes in the past did not think much about it. For most, the infection was something they just accepted, something to be endured, something that would eventually go away. They found no reason to discuss it with others, and may not have known what it was or that it might be contagious.

Then came the extensive media coverage in the late 1970s and early 1980s. The popular press turned those so affected into "lepers": harbingers of a contagious disease, and a sexually transmitted one at that. Even those with mild cases reported feeling depressed, isolated, repugnant, and contaminated, and for some there was a decreased interest in sex (Drob & Bernard, 1986).

Since genital herpes usually makes its first appearance in those 20 to 30 years of age, it can have a critical impact on sexual activity and intimacy. Being contagious and incurable, it can be disruptive to the forming of interpersonal relationships. For those who are not married, this can be a particular burden; they may feel like social outcasts, fearing that no one would want to have an intimate relationship with them, and being concerned about the ethical issues of "if, whom, and when to tell." Even before the AIDS scare, many who did not have herpes themselves, upon learning about the condition, began to restrict their own sexual experiences. To avoid contracting the infection, they stayed with partners they already knew, or limited new sexual encounters, often shunning those they learned were infected with the virus.

In the mid 1980s the AIDS outbreak quickly replaced herpes in the popular press, yet the attention previously drawn to the condition still creates practical as well as psychological problems. On one hand, those with herpes are glad to be out of the limelight; on the other hand, they often do not know where to go for help. Medically they have an incurable infection, a sexually transmittable disease. Since herpes is not as devastating as AIDS, would their concerns now be taken seriously? Would they be treated as outcasts by a public now wary of anyone whose life-style suggested even the slightest hint of promiscuity? Some have turned to support groups, called HELP, in their local communities. Here they find others with similar problems, and form a new social circle with those so affected. Some turn to psychotherapy, either individual or group, and others receive counsel from physicians.

7.2.3. Psychological Factors

Why herpes recurs is unknown, although psychological factors have been suspected as triggering mechanisms (Goldmeier & Johnson, 1982; Levenson et al., 1987; Rabkin & Struening, 1976; Silver, Auerbach, Vishniavsky, & Kaplowitz, 1986).

Silver et al. (1986) examined the relationship between psychological factors and the rate, duration, and severity (pain and bother) associated with recurrences of genital herpes infection. The men and women included in the study had severe infections, with the average recurrence rate being 9.9 per year, lasting on average 7.2 days. The sample was predominantly heterosexual (92%), Caucasian (88%), with a mean age of 33 years (range 20–65), characterized as well educated, middle to upper-middle class.

In general, the study found that persons suffering from severe cases of genital herpes show high levels of emotional dysfunction (e.g., depression, anxiety, and hostility). Exposure to stressful life events was found to be related to the duration of an outbreak, but not to the frequency of recurrence. No significant differences were reported between men and women on frequency of occurrence, duration, or bother. Women, however, rated their recurrences as more painful and were more likely to seek psychological help.

The authors concluded that the current high level of psychological distress stems primarily from the uncontrollable and unpredictable nature of the disease, the discomfort of the symptoms, and the possibility of infecting sexual partners. The subjects greatest fears involved dating and sexuality. Those with more frequent recurrences tended to view their condition as beyond their control (external locus of control) and tended to use emotion-focused, avoidant wishful thinking to cope with the distress of their condition.

Drob and Bernard (1986) used time-limited psychotherapy groups to help patients manage stress associated with genital herpes. Three groups utilized cognitive–behavioral approaches, including assertiveness training, rational emotive therapy, and neuromuscular relaxation techniques. Three other comparison groups used a structured, brief psychodynamic approach to explore issues and conflicts related to sexuality, intimacy, interpersonal relations, feelings of guilt, and self-concept. Unfortunately, the authors do not present any quantitative data regarding the differential effects of the group treatments. They anecdotally describe the effects of group treatment in general, seeing it as relieving feelings of isolation, challenging the use of denial as a defense, and exploring developmental issues that begin to emerge. They emphasize the benefits of educating patients about their illness through the exchange of information, and encouraging them to explore new ideas and behaviors in trying to adjust to the social and ethical decisions they must face.

References

Abel, G.G., Becker, J.V., Cunningham-Rathner, J., Mittelman, M., & Primack, M. Differential diagnosis of impotence in diabetes: The validity of sexual symptomatology. *Neurology and Urodynamics*, 1982, *1*, 57–69.

Abend, S.M. Serious illness in the analyst: Countertransference considerations. *Journal of the American Psychoanalytic Association*, 1982, *30*, 365–374.

Abram, H.S. Survival by machine: The psychological stress of chronic hemodialysis. In C.A. Garfield (Ed.), *Psychosocial care of the dying patient*. New York: McGraw-Hill, 1978.

Abram, H.S., Moore, G.L., & Westervelt, F.B. Suicidal behavior in chronic dialysis patients. *American Journal of Psychiatry*, 1971, *127*, 1199–1204.

Abrams, R.D. The patient with cancer: His changing patterns of communication. *New England Journal of Medicine*, 1966, *274*, 317–322.

Ader, R. (Ed.). *Psychoneuroimmunology*. New York: Academic Press, 1981.

Affleck, G., Tennen, H., Croog, S. & Levine, S. Causal attribution, perceived benefits, and morbidity after a heart attack: An 8-year study. *Journal of Consulting and Clinical Psychology*, 1987, *55*(1), 29–35.

Agle, D.P., & Baum, G.L. Psychological aspects of chronic obstructive pulmonary disease. *Medical Clinics of North America*, 1977, *61*, 749–758.

Aiken, L.H. Evaluation research and public policy: Lessons from the National Hospice Study. *Journal of Chronic Diseases*, 1986, *39*(1), 1–4.

Alexander, F. *Psychosomatic medicine*. New York: Norton, 1950.

American Cancer Society. *For men only: What you should know about prostate cancer*. New York: Author, 1981.

American Cancer Society. *Cancer facts and figures*. New York: Author, 1986.

American Psychiatric Association. *Diagnostic and statistical manual of mental disorders* (3rd ed.). Washington, DC: Author, 1980.

American Psychological Association. *A hospital practice primer for psychologists*. Washington, DC: Author, 1985.

Andersen, B.L., & Hacker, N.F. Psychosexual adjustment following pelvic exenteration. *Obstetrics and Gynecology*, 1983, *61*, 331–338. (a)

Andersen, B.L., & Hacker, N.F. Psychosexual adjustment after vulvar surgery. *Obstetrics and Gynecology*, 1983, *62*, 457–462. (b)

Andersen, B.L., & Jochimsen, P.R. Sexual functioning among breast cancer, gynecologic cancer, and healthy women. *Journal of Consulting and Clinical Psychology*, 1985, *53*(1), 25–32.

Andersen, B.L., & Jochimsen, P.R. Research design and strategy for studying psychological adjustment to cancer: Reply to Thomas. *Journal of Consulting and Clinical Psychology*, 1987, *55*(1), 122–124.

Anderson, B.J., & Wolf, F.M. Chronic physical illness and sexual behavior: Psychological issues. *Journal of Consulting and Clinical Psychology*, 1986, *54*(2), 168–175.

Andrew, J.M. Recovery from surgery, with and without preparatory instruction, for three coping styles. *Journal of Personality and Social Psychology*, 1970, *15*, 223–226.

Andrykowski, M.A., & Redd, W.H. Development of anticipatory nausea: A prospective analysis. *Journal of Consulting and Clinical Psychology*, 1985, *53*(4), 447–454.

Andrykowski, M.A., & Redd, W.H. Longitudinal analysis of the development of anticipatory nausea. *Journal of Consulting and Clinical Psychology*, 1987, *55*(1), 36–41.

Aneshensel, C.S., Frerichs, R.R., & Huba, G.J. Depression and physical illness: A multiwave, nonrecursive causal model. *Journal of Social Behavior*, 1984, *25*, 350–371.

Angell, M. Disease as a reflection of the psyche. *New England Journal of Medicine*, 1985, *312*(24), 1570–1572.

Aveline, M.O., McCulloch, D.K., Tattersall, R.B. The practice of group psychotherapy with adult-insulin dependent diabetics. *Diabetes Medicine*, 1985, *2*, 275–282.

Backman, M. The post-polio patient: Psychological issues. *Journal of Rehabilitation*, 1987, *53*(4), 23–26.

Backman, M.E., & Kopf, A.W. Iatrogenic effects of general anesthesia in children: Considerations in treating large congenital nevocytic nevi. *Journal of Dermatologic Surgery and Oncology*, 1986, *12*(4), 363–367.

Baider, L., Amikam, J.C., & Kaplan De-Nour, A. Time-limited thematic group with post-mastectomy patients. *Journal of Psychosomatic Research*, 1984, *28*(4), 323–336.

Baker, G.H.B. Psychological factors and immunity. *Journal of Psychosomatic Research*, 1987, *31*(1), 1–10.

Barefoot, J.C., Dahlstrom, W.G., & Williams, R.B. Hostility, CHD incidence, and total mortality: A 25-year follow-up study of 255 physicians. *Psychosomatic Medicine*, 1983, *45*(1), 59–63.

Barsky, A., & Klerman, G. Overview: Hypochondriasis, bodily complaints and somatic styles. *American Journal of Psychiatry*, 1983, *140*, 273–283.

Barsky, A., & Klerman, G. Hypochondrias. *Harvard Medical School Mental Health Letter*, 1985, *2*(6), 4–6.

Bartrop, R.W., Lazarus, L., Luckhurst, E., Kiloh, L.G., & Penny, R. Depressed lymphocyte function after bereavement. *Lancet*, 1977, *1*, 834–836.

Battin, M.P. The concept of rational suicide. In M.P. Battin, *Ethical issues in suicide*. Englewood Cliffs, NJ: Prentice-Hall, 1982.

Batzel, L.W., & Dodrill, C.B. Emotional and intellectual correlatives of unsuccessful suicide attempts in people with epilepsy. *Journal of Clinical Psychology*, 1986, *42*(5), 699–702.

Bean, G., Cooper, S., Alpert, R., & Kipnis, D. Coping mechanisms of cancer patients: A study of 33 patients receiving chemotherapy. *CA—A Cancer Journal for Clinicians*, 1980, *30*, 256–259.

Bear, D., Fedio, P. Quantitative analysis of interictal behavior in temporal lobe epilepsy. *Archives of Neurology*, 1977, *34*, 454–469.

Beck, A.T., Rush, A.J., Shaw, B.F., & Emery, G. *Cognitive therapy of depression*, New York: Guilford Press, 1979.

Belgrave, F.Z., & Washington, A. The relationship between locus of control and select personality traits in two chronically ill adolescent patient groups. *Journal of Rehabilitation*, 1986, *533*(4), 57–60.

Bennett, P., & Wilkinson, S. A comparison of psychological and medical treatment of the irritable bowel syndrome. *British Journal of Clinical Psychology*, 1985, *24*, 215–216.

Berkman, L., & Syme, S. Social networks, host resistance and mortality: A nine-year follow-up study of Alameda County residents. *American Journal of Epidemiology*, 1979, *109*, 186–204.

Beutler, L.E., Engle, D., Oro'-Beutler, M.E., Daldrup, R., & Meredith, K. Inability to express intense affect: A common link between depression and pain? *Journal of Consulting and Clinical Psychology*, 1986, *54*(6), 752–759.

Bexton, W., Heron, W., & Scott, T. Effects of decreased variation in the sensory environment. *Canadian Journal of Psychology*, 1954, *8*, 70–76.

Binger, C.M., Ablin, A.R., Feuerstein, R.C., Kushner, J.H., Zoger, S., & Mikkelsen, C. Childhood leukemia: Emotional impact on patient and family. *New England Journal of Medicine*, 1969, *280*, 414–418.

Binik, Y.M. Coping with chronic life-threatening illness: Psychosocial perspectives on end stage renal disease. *Canadian Journal of Behavioural Science*, 1983, *15*(4), 373–391.

Blackburn, S.L. Dietary compliance of chronic hemodialysis patients. *Journal of Consulting and Clinical Psychology*, 1977, *70*, 31–37.

Block, J. Herpes: Scourge of the seventies. *Canadian Nurse*, 1980, *1*, 22–24.

Blumenthal, J.A., Burg, M.M., Barefoot, J., Williams, R.B., Haney, T., & Zimet, G. Social support, Type A behavior, and coronary artery disease. *Psychosomatic Medicine*, 1987, *49*, 331–340.

Blumer, D. Epilepsy and its psychiatric dimension. *Harvard Medicine School Mental Health Letter*, 1986, *2*(7), 4–5.

Boehnert, C.E., & Popkin, M.K. Psychological issues in treatment of severely noncompliant diabetics. *Psychosomatics*, 1986, *27*(1), 11–20.

Bowman, J.T. Attitudes toward disabled persons: Social distance and work competence. *Journal of Rehabilitation*, 1987, *53*(1), 41–44.

Bozarth, C.H. Unfinished business: *Some feelings surrounding the late effects of polio*. Okemos, MI: Polio Survivors' Support Group of Lansing, March 1987.

Brent, D.A. Overrepresentation of epileptics in a consecutive series of suicide attempters seen at a children's hospital, 1978–1983. *Journal of the American Academy of Child Psychiatry*, 1986, *25*(2), 242–246.

Brook, B.N. Dyspareunia: A significant symptom in Crohn's disease. *Lancet*, 1979, *1*, 1199.

Brooks, G.R., & Richardson, F.C. Emotional skills training: A treatment program for duodenal ulcer. *Behavior Therapy*, 1980, *11*, 198–207.

Brown, J.H., Henteleff, P., Barakat, S., & Rowe, C.J. Is it normal for terminally ill patients to desire death? *American Journal of Psychiatry*, 1986, *143*(2), 208–211.

Brownlee-Duffeck, M., Peterson, L., Simonds, J.F., Goldstein, D., Kilo, C., & Hoette, S. The role of health beliefs in the regimen adherence and metabolic control of adolescents and adults with diabetes mellitus. *Journal of Consulting and Clinical Psychology*, 1987, *55*(2), 139–144.

Bruno, R.L., & Frick, N.M. Stress and "Type A" behavior as precipitants of post-polio sequelae: The Felician/Columbia Survey. In L.S. Halstead & D.O. Wiechers (Eds.), *Research and clinical aspects of the late effects of poliomyelitis*. White Plains, NY: March of Dimes Birth Defects Foundation, 1987.

Bucher, J., Smith, E., & Gillespie, C. Short-term group therapy for stroke patients in a rehabilitation centre. *British Journal of Medical Psychology*, 1984, *57*, 283–290.

Bukberg, J. Penman, D., & Holland, J.C. Depression in hospitalized cancer patients. *Psychosomatic Medicine*, 1984, *46*(3), 199–212.

Burish, T.G., & Bradley, L.A. Coping with chronic disease: Definitions and issues. In T.G. Burish & L.A. Bradley (Eds.), *Copying with chronic disease: Research and applications*. New York: Academic Press, 1983.

Burish, T.G., & Carey, M.P. Conditioned responses to cancer chemotherapy: Etiology and treatment. In B.H. Fox & B.H. Newberry (Eds.), *Impact of psychoendocrine systems in cancer and immunity* (pp. 147–178). Toronto: C.J. Hogrefe, 1984.

Burish, T.G., Carey, M.P., Krozely, M.G., & Greco, F.A. Conditioned side effects induced by cancer chemotherapy: Prevention through behavioral treatment. *Journal of Consulting and Clinical Psychology*, 1987, *15*(1), 42–48.

Burish, T.G., & Lyles, J.N. Coping with the adverse effects of cancer treatments. In T.G. Burish & L.A. Bradley (Eds.), *Copying with chronic disease: Research and applications*. New York: Academic Press, 1983.

Burish, T.B., Shartner, C.D., & Lyles, J.N. Effectiveness of multiple-site EMG biofeedback and relaxation in reducing the aversiveness of cancer chemotherapy. *Biofeedback and Self-Regulation*, 1981, *6*, 523–535.

Burr, B.B., Good, J.B., & Del Veccio-Good, M. The impact of illness on the family. In R.B. Taylor (Ed.), *Family medicine: Principles and practice*. New York: Springer-Verlag, 1978, pp. 221–233.

Caldwell, H.S., & Leveque, K.L. Group psychotherapy in the management of hemophilia. *Psychological Reports*, 1974, *35*, 339.

Campbell, I.W., & McCulloch, D.K. Marital problems in diabetics. *Practitioner*, 1979, *222*, 343–347.

Caplan, L.M. Pre-education of the potentially blind as a deterrent to suicide. *Psychosomatics*, 1981, *22*(2), 165, 169.

Carey, M.P., & Burish, T.G. Anxiety as a predictor of behavioral therapy outcome for cancer chemotherapy patients. *Journal of Consulting and Clinical Psychology*, 1985, *53*(6), 860–865.

Case, R.B., Heller, S.S., Case. N.B., Moss, A.J., & The Multicenter Post-infarction Research Group. Type A behavior and survival after acute myocardial infarction. *New England Journal of Medicine*, 1985, *312*(12), 739–741.

Cassileth, B.R., Lusk, E.J., Miller, D.S., Brown, L.L., & Miller C. Psychosocial correlates of survival in advanced malignant disease. *New England Journal of Medicine*, 1985, *312*, 1551–1555.

Cassileth, B.R., Lusk, E.J., Strouse, T.B., Miller, D.S., Brown, L.L., Cross, P.A., Tenaglia, A.N. Psychological status in chronic illness: A comparative analysis of six diagnostic groups. *New England Journal of Medicine*, 1984, *311*(8), 506–511.

Cassileth, B.R., Zupkis, R.V., Sutton-Smith, K., & March, V. Information and participation preferences among cancer patients. *Annals of Internal Medicine*, 1980, *92*, 832–836.

Cella, D.F., & Tross S. Psychological adjustment to survival from Hodgkin's disease. *Journal of Consulting and Clinical Psychology*, 1986, *54*(5), 616–622.

Chalon, J., Hillman, D., Gross, S., Eisner, M., Tang, C., & Turndorf, H., Interuterine exposure to halothane increases murine postnatal autotolerance to halothane and reduces brain weight. *Anesthesiology Analogs*, 1983, *62*, 565–567.

Chalon, J., Tang, C., Ramanathan, S., Eisner, M., Katz, R., & Turndorf, H. Exposure to halothane and enflurane affects learning function of murine progency. *Anesthesiology Analogs*, 1981, *60*, 794–797.

Chernin, P. Illness in a therapist: Loss of omnipotence. *Archives of General Psychiatry*, 1976, *33*, 1327–1328.

Chesney, M.A., & Rosenman, R.H. (Eds.). *Anger and hostility in cardiovascular and behavioral disorders*. New York: Hemisphere, 1985.

Chubon, R.A. Group practices in the rehabilitation of physically disabled persons. In M. Seligman (Ed.), *Group psychotherapy and counselling with special populations*. Baltimore: University Park Press, 1982.

Clark, D.C., Cavanaugh, S.V., & Gibbons, R.D. The core symptoms of depression in medical and psychiatric patients. *Journal of Nervous and Mental Disease*, 1983, *171*, 705–713.

Clark, R., Hailstone, J.D., & Slade, P.D. Psychological aspects of dialysis: A semantic differential study. *Psychological Medicine*, 1979, *9*, 55–62.

Cohen, S., & Matthews, K.A. Social support, Type A behavior, and coronary artery disease. *Psychosomatic Medicine*, 1978, *49*, 325–330.

Colorez, A., & Geist, G.O. Rehabilitation vs. general employer attitudes toward hiring disabled persons. *Journal of Rehabilitation*, 1987, *53*(2), 44–47.

Conte, H.R., & Karasu, T.B. Psychotherapy for medically ill patients: Review and critique of controlled studies. *Psychosomatics*, 1981, *22*, 285–315.

Corey, I., Adams, E.G., Brown, Z.A., & Holmes, K.K. Genital herpes simplex virus infections: Clinical manifestations, course, and implications. *Internal Medicine*, 1983, *98*, 958–972.

Cox, D.J., Gonder-Frederick, L., Pohl, S., & Pennebaker, J.W. Diabetes. In K.A. Holroyd & T.L. Creer (Eds.), *Self-management of chronic disease: Handbook of clinical interventions and research*. New York: Academic Press, 1986.

Creer, T. Asthma: Psychological aspects and management. In E. Middleton, C. Reed, & E. Ellis (Eds.), *Allergy: Principles and practice*, St. Louis, MO: Mosby, 1978.

Creer, T. Asthma. *Journal of Consulting and Clinical Psychology*, 1982, *50*, 912–921.

Cronkite, R.C., & Moos, R.H. The role of predisposing and moderating factors in the stress–illness relationship. *Journal of Health and Social Behavior*, 1984, *25*(December), 372–393.

Cummings, K.M., Becker, H.H., Kirscht, J.P., & Levin, N.W. Intervention strategies to improve compliance with medical regimens by ambulatory hemodialysis patients. *Journal of Behavioral Medicine*, 1981, *4*, 111–127.

Daly, M.J. Psychological impact of surgical procedures on women. In B.J. Saddock, H.I. Kaplan, & A.M. Freedman (Eds.), *The sexual experience*. Baltimore: Williams & Wilkins, 1976.

Davis, F. *Passage through crisis: Polio victims and their families.* Indianapolis: Bobbs-Merrill, 1963.

Davis, M., Eshelman, E.R., & McKay, M. *The relaxation and stress reduction workbook.* Richmond, CA: New Harbinger Publications, 1980.

Davis, L.G., & Kenney, R.E. Genital herpes simplex virus infection: Clinical course and attempted therapy. *American Journal of Hospital Pharmacy*, 1981, *38*, 825–829.

DeLeon, P.H., Uyeda, M.K., & Welch, B.L. Psychology and HMOs: New partnership or new adversary. *American Psychologist*, 1985, *40*(10), 1122–1124.

Dell Orto, A., & Laskey, E. Group counseling and physical disability. North Scituate, MA: Duxbury Press, 1979.

Dembroski, T.J., & McDougall, J.M. Stress, emotions, behavior and cardiovascular disease. In C. Van Dyke, L. Temoschak, & L. Segans (Eds.), *Emotions in health and illness* (Vol. 1). San Diego: Grune and Stratton, 1983.

Dennerstein, L., Wood, C., & Burrows, G.D. Sexual response following hysterectomy and oophorectomy. *Obstetrics and Gynecology*, 1977, *49*, 92–97.

Derogatis, L.R. Breast and gynecologic cancers: Their unique impact on body image and sexual identity in women. In J.M. Vaeth (Ed.), *Frontiers of radiation therapy and oncology* (Vol. 14). Basel, Switzerland: Karger, 1980, (pp. 1–11).

Derogatis, L.R. The Psychosocial Adjustment to Illness Scale (PAIS). *Journal of Psychosomatic Research*, 1986, *30*(1), 77–91.

Derogatis, L.R., Abeloff, M.D., & McBeth, C.D. Cancer patients and their physicians in the perception of psychological symptoms. *Psychosomatic*, 1976, *17*, 197–201.

Derogatis, L.R., Abeloff, M.D., & Melisaratos, N., Psychological coping mechanisms and survival time in metastatic breast cancer. *Journal of the American Medical Association*, 1979, *242*, 1504–1508.

Dewald, P.A. Serious illness in the analyst: Transference, countertransference, and reality responses. *Journal of the American Psychoanalytic Association*, 1982, *30*, 347–363.

Dilley, J.W., Shelp, E.E., & Batki, S.L. Psychiatric and ethical issues in the care of patients with AIDS. *Psychosomatics*, 1986, *27*(8), 562–566.

Dimsdale, J.E. A perspective on Type A behavior and coronary disease. *New England Journal of Medicine*, 1988, *318*(2), 110–112.

Dorpat, T.L. Anderson, W.F., & Ripley, H.S. The relationship of physical illness to suicide. In H.L. Resnik (Ed.), *Suicidal behaviors: Diagnosis and management*. Boston: Little, Brown, 1968.

Drob, S., & Bernard, H.S. Time-limited group treatment of genital herpes patients. *International Journal of Group Psychotherapy*, 1986, *36*(1), 133–144.

Druss, R.G. Psychotherapy of patients with serious intercurrent medical illness (cancer). *Journal of the American Academy of Psychoanalysis*, 1986, *14*(4), 459–472.

Dumas, R.G., & Leonard, R.C. The effect of nursing on the incidence of postoperative vomiting. *Nursing Research*, 1963, *12*, 12–15.

Dunkel-Schetter, C. Social support and cancer: Findings based on patient interviews and their implications. *Journal of Social Issues*, 1984, *40*, 77–98.

Earl, W.L. Job stability and family counseling. *Epilepsia*, 1986, *27*(3), 215–219.

Egbert, L., Battit, G., Welch, C., & Bartlett, M. Reduction of post-operative pain by encouragement and instruction of patients. *New England Journal of Medicine*, 1964, *270*, 825–827.

Eissler, K.R. On the possible effects of aging on the practice of psychoanalysis. *Psychoanalytic Quarterly*, 1977, *46*, 182–183.

Epilepsy Foundation of America. *Questions and answers about epilepsy*. Landover, MD: Author, 1982.

Epilepsy Foundation of America. *Epilepsy: Recognition and first aid*. Landover, MD: Author, 1983.

Epilepsy Foundation of America. *Medications for epilepsy*. Landover, MD.: Author, 1985.

Erickson, E.H. *Identity and the life cycle*. New York: International Universities Press, 1959.

Evans, D.L., McCartney, C.F., Nemeroff, C.B., Raft, D., Quade, D., Golden, R.N., Haggerty, J.J., Holmes, V., Simon, J.S., Droba, M., Mason, G.A., & Fowler, W.C. Depression in women treated for gynecological cancer: Clinical and neuroendocrine assessment. *American Journal of Psychiatry*, 1986, *143*(6), 447–452.

Farberow, N.L. Suicide prevention in the hospital. *Hospital and Community Psychiatry*, 1981, *32*(2), 99–104.

Farberow, N.L. Ganzler, S., Cutter, F., & Reynolds, D. An eight-year survey of hospital suicides, *Life-Threatening Behaviour*, 1971, *1*(3), 184–202.

Farberow, N.L, McKelligott, J.W., Cohen, S., & Darbonne, A. Suicide among patients with cardiorespiratory illnesses. *Journal of the American Medical Association*, 1966, *195*, 128–134.

Farberow, N.L., Shneidman, E.S., & Leonard, C.V. Suicide among general medical and surgical hospital patients and those with malignant neoplasms. *Medical Bulletin of the Veterans Administration*, 1963, *9*, 1–11.

Ferlic, M., Goldman, A., & Kennedy, B.J. Group counseling in adult patients with advanced cancer. *Cancer*, 1979, *43*, 760–766.

Fink, R., & Shapiro, S. Patterns of medical care related to mental illness. *Journal of Health and Human Behavior*, 1966, *7*, 98–105.

Fischer, A.B. Knop, J. & Graem, N. Late mortality following Billroth II resection for duodenal ulcer. *Acta Chirurgica Scandinavica*, 1985, *151*(1), 43–47.

Fischman, J. Type A on trial. *Psychology Today*, February 1987, pp. 42–50.

Fisher, K. Health psychology. *APA Monitor*, January 1986, pp. 16–17.

Flaherty, J.A. Self-disclosure in therapy: Marriage of the therapist. *American Journal of Psychotherapy*, 1979, *33*(3), 442–451.

Flavin, D.K., Franklin, J.E., & Frances, R.J. The acquired immune deficiency syndrome (AIDS) and suicidal behavior in alcohol-dependent homosexual men. *American Journal of Psychiatry*, 1986, *143*(11), 1440–1442.

Follette, W., & Cummings, N.A. Psychiatric services and medical utilization in a prepaid health plan setting. *Medical Care*, 1967, *5*, 25–35.

Frances, R.J., Wikstrom, T., & Alcena, V. Contracting AIDS as a means of committing suicide (letter). *American Journal of Psychiatry*, 1985, *142*, 656.

Freidenbergs, I. Psychosocial management of patients with cutaneous cancers: A preliminary report. *Journal of Dermatologic Surgery and Oncology*, 1981, *7*(10), 828–830.

Freidenbergs, I., Gordon, W., Hibbard, M., Levine, L., Wolf, C., & Diller, L. Psychosocial aspects of living with cancer: A review of the literature. *International Journal of Psychiatry in Medicine*, 1981–1982, *11*(4), 303–329.

French, D.J., McDowell, R.E., and Keith, R.A. Participant observation as a patient in a rehabilitation hospital. *Rehabilitation Psychology*, 1971, *19*, 89–95.

Frick, N.M., & Bruno, R.L. Post-polio sequelae: Physiological and psychological overview. *Rehabilitation Literature*, 1986, *47*(5–6), 106–111.

Friedman, H.S., & Booth-Kewley, S. The "disease-prone personality": A meta-analytic view of the construct. *American Psychologist*, 1987, *42*(6), 539–555.

Friedman, M., Thoresen, C., Gill, J., Powell, L., Ulmer, D., Thompson, L., Price, V.A., Rabin, D.D., Breall, W.S., Dixon, T., Levy, R., & Bourg, E. Alteration of Type A behavior and reduction in cardiac occurrences in postmyocardial infarction patients. *American Heart Journal*, 1984, *108*(2), 237–248.

Friis, M.L. Epilepsy among parents of children with facial clefts. *Epilepsia*, 1979, *20*, 69–76.

Fromm-Reichmann, F. *Principles of intensive psychotherapy*. Chicago: University of Chicago Press, 1950.

Gabriel, H.P. A practical approach to preparing children for dermatology surgery. *Journal of Dermatologic Surgery and Oncology*, 1977, *3*, 523–526.

Garfield, C.A. (Ed.). *Psychosocial care of the dying patient*. New York: McGraw-Hill, 1978.

Garfield, J.M. Psychologic problems in anesthesia. *American Family Physician*, 1974, *10*(2), 60–67.

Garrity, T.F. Social involvement and activeness as predictors of morale six months after myocardial infarction. *Social Science Medicine*, 1973, *7*, 199–207. (a)

Garrity, T.F. Vocational adjustment after first myocardial infarction: Comparative assessment of several variables suggested in the literature. *Social Science and Medicine*, 1973, *7*, 705–717. (b)

Garrity, T.F. Morbidity, mortality and rehabilitation. In W.D. Gentry & R.B. Williams, Jr. (Eds.), *Psychological aspects of myocardial infarction and coronary care*. St. Louis, Mo.: C.V. Mosby, 1975.

Geisler, W.O., Jousse, A.T., Wynne-Jones, M., & Breithaupt, D. Survival in traumatic spinal cord injury. *Paraplegia*, 1983, *21*, 364–373.

Geringer, E.S., & Stern, T.A. Coping with medical illness: The impact of personality types. *Psychosomatics*, 1986, *27*(4), 251–261.

Gilman, A.G., Goodman, L.S., & Gilman, A. (Eds)., *Goodman and Gilman's The Pharmacological basis of therapeutics* (6th ed.). New York: Macmillan, 1980.

Givelber, F., & Simon B. A death in the life of a therapist and its impact on the therapy. *Psychiatry*, 1981, *44*, 141–149.

Goldberg, J.D., Krantz, G., & Locke, B.Z. Effect of a short-term outpatient psychiatric therapy benefit on utilization of medical services in a prepaid group practice medical program. *Medical Care*, 1970, *8*, 419–428.

Goldmeier, D., & Johnson, A. Does psychiatric illness affect the recurrence rate of genital herpes? *British Journal of Venereal Disease*, 1982, *58*, 40–43.

Goldwyn, R.M. (Ed.) *The unfavorable result in plastic surgery: Avoidance and treatment* (2nd ed.). Boston: Little Brown, 1984.

Goodkin, K., Antoni, M.H., & Blaney, P.H. Stress and hopelessness in the promotion of cervical intraepithelial neoplasis to invasive squamous cell carcinoma of the cervix. *Journal of Psychosomatic Research*, 1986, *30*, 67–76.

Gordon, W.A., Freidenbergs, I., Diller, L., Hibbard, M., Wolf, C., Levine, L., Lipkins, R., Ezrachi, O., & Lucido, D. Efficacy of psychosocial intervention with cancer patients. *Journal of Consulting and Clinical Psychology*, 1980, *48*, 743–759.

Gots, R., & Kaufman, A. *The people's hospital book*. New York: Avon, 1981.

Graham, S. Alcohol and breast cancer. *New England Journal of Medicine*, 1987, *316*(19), 1174–1180.

Grant, D., & Anns, M. Counseling AIDS antibody-positive clients: Reactions and treatment. *American Psychologist*, 1988, *43*(1), 72–74.

Grant, W.W. What parents of a chronically ill or dysfunctioning child always want to know but may be afraid to ask. *Clinical Pediatrics*, 1978, *17*, 915–917.

Green, J.A., & Shellenberger, R.D. Biofeedback research and the ghost in the box: A reply to Roberts. *American Psychologist*, 1986, *41*, 1003–1005.

Green, J.B., & Mercille, R.A. Psychiatric complications of epilepsy. *Neurologic Clinics*, 1984, *2*(1), 103–112.

Greenfield, S., Blanco, D.M., Elashoff, R.M., & Ganz, P.A. Patterns of care related to age of breast cancer patients. *Journal of the American Medical Association*, 1987, *257*(20), 2766–2770.

Greer, D.S., & Mor, V. An overview of National Hospice Study findings. *Journal of Chronic Diseases*, 1986, *39*(1), 5–7.

Greer, D.S., Mor, V., Morris, J.N., Sherwood, S., Kidder, D., & Birnbaum, H. An alternative in terminal care: Results of the National Hospice Study. *Journal of Chronic Diseases*, 1986, *39*(1), 9–26.

Grossman, J.H., Wallen, W.C., & Sever, J.L. Management of genital herpes simplex virus infection during pregnancy. *Obstetrics and Gynecology*, 1981, *58*, 1–4.

Gruen, W. Effects of brief psychotherapy during the hospitalization period on the recovery process in heart attacks. *Journal of Consulting and Clinical Psychology*, 1975, *43*, 223–232.

Gurrister, L., & Kane, R.A. How therapists perceive and treat suicidal patients. *Community Mental Health Journal*, 1978, *14*(1), 3–13.

Halligan, F.R., & Reznikoff, M. Personality factors and change with multiple sclerosis. *Journal of Consulting and Clinical Psychology*, 1985, *53*(4), 547–548.

Halpert, E. When the analyst is chronically ill. *Psychoanalytic Quarterly*. 1982, *51*, 372–389.

Halstead, L., & Wiechers, D. (Eds.). *Late effects of poliomyelitis*. Miami: Symposia Foundation, 1985.

Halstead, L.S., & Wiechers, D.O. (Eds.). *Research and clinical aspects of the late effects of poliomyelitis*. White Plains, NY: March of Dimes Birth Defects Foundation, 1987.

Hansen, L.C., & McAleer, C.A. Terminal cancer and suicide: The health care professional's dilemma. *Omega*, 1983–1984, *14*(3), 241–248.

Harris, L.L., Vogtsberger, K.N., & Mattox, D.E. Group psychotherapy for head and neck cancer patients. *Laryngoscope*, 1985, *95*, 585–587.

Hartz, J. Tuberculosis and personality conflicts. *Psychosomatic Medicine*, 1944, *6*, 17–22.

Hartz, J. Human relationships in tuberculosis. *Public Health Report*, 1950, *65*, 1292–1305.

Hawton, K., Fagg, J., & Marsack, P. Association between epilepsy and attempted suicide. *Journal of Neurology, Neurosurgery and Psychiatry*, 1980, *43*, 163–170.

Hayes, J.R., Butler, N.E., & Martin, C.R. Misunderstood somatopsychic concomitants of medical disorders. *Psychosomatics*, 1986, *27*(2), 128–133.

Haynes, R.B., Taylor, D.W., & Sackett, D.L. (Eds.). *Compliance in health care*. Baltimore: Johns Hopkins University Press, 1979.

Heinrich, R.L., & Schag, C.C. The psychosocial impact of cancer: Cancer patients and healthy controls (Report No. 85-105). Sepulveda, CA: Sepulveda VA Medical Center, Behavioral Rehabilitation Research Department, 1985. (a)

Heinrich, R.L., & Schag, C.C. Stress and activity management: Group treatment for cancer patients and spouses. *Journal of Consulting and Clinical Psychology*, 1985, *53*(4), 439–446. (b)

Heller, S., & Kornfeld, D. Delirium and related problems. In S. Arieti (Ed.), *American handbook of psychiatry* (2nd ed., Vol. 4), 1975, pp. 45–66. New York: Basic Books.

Heller, V. Handicapped patients talk together. *Journal of Nursing*, 1970, *70*, 332–335.

Henriques, B., Stadil, F., & Baden, H. Patient information about cancer: A prospective study of patients' opinion and reaction to information about cancer diagnosis. *Acta Chirurgica Scandinavica*, 1980, *146*, 309–311.

Hermann, B.P., & Chhabria, S. Interictal psychopathology in patients with ictal fear: Examples of sensorary-limbic hyperconnection? *Archives of Neurology*, 1980, *37*, 667–668.

Hermann, B.P., Schwartz, M.S., Whitman, S., & Karnes, W.E. Aggression and epilepsy: Seizure-type comparisons and high-risk variables. *Epilepsia*, 1980, *22*, 691–698.

Hertz, S.M., Greenberg, R., & Baredes, S. The role of the psychiatrist in otolaryngology. *Otolaryngologic Clinics of North America*, 1984, *17*(4), 735–743.

Hoban, P. The surgeon's helping hand. *New York Magazine*, November 1984, pp. 30–31.

Holland, J. Psychological aspects of oncology. *Medical Clinics of North America*, 1977, *61*(4), 737–748.

Holland, J.C., Korzun, A.H., Tross, S., Silberfarb, P., Perry, M., Comis, R., & Oster, M. Comparative psychological disturbance in patients with pancreatic and gastric cancer. *American Journal of Psychiatry*, 1986, *143*(8), 982–986.

Holland, J.D., & Mastrovito, R. Psychologic adaption to breast cancer. *Cancer*, 1980, *46*, 1045–1052.

Holmes, T.H., Hawkins, N.G., Bowerman, C.E., Clarke, E.R., & Joffe, J.R. Psychosocial and psychophysiologic studies of tuberculosis. *Psychosomatic Medicine*, 1957, *19*, 134–143.

Holroyd, K. Recurrent headache. In K.A. Holroyd & T.L. Creer (Eds.), *Self-management of chronic disease: Handbook of clinical interventions and research*. New York: Academic Press, 1986.

Horne, R.L., & Picard, R.S. Psychosocial risk factors for lung cancer. *Psychosomatic Medicine*, 1979, *41*, 503–514.

Horowitz, J. Polio's painful legacy. *New York Times Sunday Magazine*, July 7, 1985, pp. 16–23.

Houston, B.K., & Kelly, K.E. Type A behavior in housewives: Relation to work, marital adjustment, stress, tension, health, fear-of-failure and self-esteem. *Journal of Psychosomatic Research*, 1987, *31*(1) 55–61.

Huberty, D.J. Adapting to illness through family group. *International Journal of Psychiatry in Medicine*, 1974, *11*, 213–218.

Huchcroft, S. Suicide among cancer patients. *Eppi-Log*, 1984, *1*(4), 5–9.

Hyland, J.M., Pruyser, H., Novotny, E., & Coyne, L. The impact of the death of a group member in a group of breast cancer patients. *International Journal of Group Psychotherapy*, 1984, *34*(4), 617–626.

Ibrahim, M.A., Feldman, J.G., Sultz, H.A., Staiman, M.G., Young, I.J., & Dean, D. Management after myocardial infarction: A controlled trial of the effect of group psychotherapy. *International Journal of Psychiatry in Medicine*, 1974, *5*, 253–268.

ICD—International Center for the Disabled. *The ICD survey of disabled Americans: Bringing disabled Americans into the mainstream*. New York: Author, 1986.

ICD—International Center for the Disabled. *The ICD survey II: Employing disabled Americans*. New York: Author, 1987.

Imbus, S.H., & Zawacki, B.E. Autonomy for burn patients when survival is unprecedented. *New England Journal of Medicine*, 1977, *297*(6), 308–311.

Isler, C. Radiation therapy: 2. The nurse and the patient. *RN Magazine*, 1971, *34*, 48–51.

Jamison, K.R., Wellisch, D.K., & Pasnau, R.O. Psychosocial aspects of mastectomy, I: The woman's perspective. *American Journal of Psychiatry*, 1978, *135*, 432–436.

Jefferys, D.B., & Volans, G.N. Self-poisoning in diabetic patients. *Human Toxicology*, 1983, *2*(2), 345–348.

Jemmot, J.B., & Locke, S.E. Psychosocial factors, immunological mediation, and human susceptibility to infectious diseases: How much do we know? *Psychological Bulletin*, 1984, *95*, 78–108.

Jensen, S.B. Diabetic sexual dysfunction: A comparative study of 160 insulin treated men and women and an age-matiched control group. *Archives of Sexual Behavior*, 1981, *10*, 493–504.

Kahneman, D., & Tversky, A. Choices, values, and frames. *American Psychologist*, 1984, *39*(4), 341–350.

Kalish, R., & Reynolds, D. *Death and ethnicity: A psychological study*. Los Angeles: University of Southern California Press, 1976.

Kanas, N., Kaltreider, N., & Horowitz, M. Response to catastrophe: A case study. *Diseases of the Nervous System*, 1977, *37*(8), 625–677.

Kaplan, A.H. & Rothman, D. The dying psychotherapist. *American Journal of Psychiatry*, 1986, *143*(5), 561–572.

Kaplan, B.J., & Wyler, A.R. Coping with epilepsy. In T.G. Burish & L.A. Bradley (Eds.), *Coping with chronic disease: Research and applications*. New York: Academic Press, 1983.

Kathol, R.G., & Petty, F. Relationship of depression to medical illness: A critical review. *Journal of Affective Disorders*, 1981, *3*, 111–121.

Kellner, R. Psychotherapy in psychosomatic disorders: A survey of controlled studies. *Archives of General Psychiatry*, 1975, *32*, 1021–1028.

Khan, A.U. *Psychiatric emergencies in pediatrics*. Chicago: Year Book Publishers, 1979.

Kiecolt-Glaser, J.K., & Glaser, R. Psychological influences on immunity. *Psychosomatics*, 1986, 27(9), 621–624.

Kirkpatrick, J.R. The stoma patient and his return to society. *Frontiers of Radiation Therapy and Oncology*, 1980, 14, 20–25.

Kog, E., Vertommen, H., & Vandereycken, W. Minuchin's psychosomatic family model revised: A concept-validation study using a multitrait-multimethod approach. *Family Process*, 1987, 26, 235–253.

Kohl, S.J. Emotional responses to the late effects of poliomyelitis. In L.S. Halstead & D.O. Wiechers (Eds.), *Research and clinical aspects of the late effects of poliomyelitis*. White Plains, NY: March of Dimes Birth Defects Foundation, 1987.

Kokaska, C.J., & Maslow, P. Employment of people with epilepsy: A review of employer attitude surveys. *Journal of Rehabilitation*, 1986, 52(4), 31–33.

Kolodny, C.R. Sexual dysfunction in diabetic females. *Diabetes*, 1971, 20, 557–559.

Koocher, G.P. Coping with a death from cancer. *Journal of Consulting and Clinical Psychology*, 1986, 54(5), 623–631.

Koocher, G.P., & O'Malley, J.E. *The Damocles syndrome: Psychological consequences of surviving childhood cancer*. New York: McGraw-Hill, 1981.

Korchin, S.J. *Modern clinical psychology: Principles of intervention in the clinic and community*. New York: Basic Books, 1976.

Krantz, D.S., Baum, A., & Singer, J.E. (Eds.). *Handbook of psychology and health: Vol 3. Cardiovascular disorders and behavior*. Hillsdale, NJ: Erlbaum, 1983.

Krantz, D.S., Baum, A., & Wideman, M. Assessment of preferences for self-treatment and information in health care. *Journal of Personality and Social Psychology*, 1980, 39, 977–990.

Krantz, D.S., & Deckel, A.W. Coping with coronary heart disease and stroke. In T.G. Burish & L.A. Bradley (Eds.), *Coping with chronic disease: Research and application*. New York: Academic Press, 1983.

Kriechman, A.M. Illness in the therapist: The eye patch. *Psychiatry*, 1984, 47, 378–386.

Krosnick, A., & Podolsky, S. Diabetes and sexual dysfunction: Restoring normal ability. *Geriatrics, 36*, 1981, 92–100.

Kübler-Ross, E. *On death and dying*. London: Tavistock, 1969.

Langeluddecke, P., Goulston, K., & Tennant, C. Type A behaviour and other psychological factors in peptic ulcer disease. *Journal of Psychosomatic Research*, 1987, 31(3), 335–340.

Langer, E.J., Janis, I.L., & Wolfer, J.A. Reduction of psychological stress in surgical patients. *Journal of Experimental Social Psychology*, 1975, 11, 155–163.

Laurie, G. (Ed.). Respiratory rehabilitation and post-polio aging problems. *Rehabilitation Gazette*, 1980, 23, 3–10.

Laurie, G., Maynard, F., Fischer, D., & Raymond, J. (Eds.). *Handbook on the late effects of poliomyelitis for physicians and survivors*. St. Louis, MO: Gazette International Networking Institute, 1984.

Laurie, G., & Raymond, J. Polio support groups guidelines. *Rehabilitation Gazette*, 1985, 26, 30–35.

Lazarus, R.S. The costs and benefits of denial. In S. Breznitz (Ed.), *The denial of stress*. New York: International Universities Press, 1983.

Lazarus, R.S., & Launier, R. Stress-related transactions between person and environment. In L.A. Pervin & M. Lewis (Eds.), *Perspectives in interactional psychology*. New York: Plenum Press, 1978.

Levenson, J.L., Hamer, R.M., Myers, T., Hart, R.P., & Kaplowitz, L.G. Psychological factors predict symptoms of severe recurrent genital herpes infection. *Journal of Psychosomatic Research*, 1987, 31(2), 153–159.

Levine, P.M., Silberfarb, P.M., & Lipowski, Z.J. Mental disorders in cancer patients: A study of 100 psychiatric referrals. *Cancer*, 1978, 42, 1385–1391.

Levine, J., Warrenburg, S., Kerns, R., Schwartz, G., Delaney, R., Fontana, A., Gradman, A.,

Smith, S., Allen, S., & Cascione, R. The role of denial in recovery from coronary heart disease. *Psychosomatic Medicine*, 1987, *49*(2), 109–117.

Levitan, H. Suicidal trends in patients with asthma and hypertension. A chart study. *Psychotherapy and Psychosomantics*, 1983, *39*, 165–170.

Levy, N.B. Psychological reactions to machine dependency: Hemodialysis. *Psychiatric Clinics of North America*, 1981, *4*, 351–363.

Levy, N.B. Psychological complications of dialysis: Psychonephrology to the rescue. *Bulletin of the Menninger Clinic*, 1984, *48*(3), 237–250.

Levy, N.B., & Wyntraub, G.D. The quality of life on maintenance hemodialysis. *Lancet*, 1975, *1*, 1328–1330.

Levy, R.M., Pons, V.G., & Rosenblum, M.L. Central nervous system mass lesions in the acquired immune deficiency syndrome (AIDS). *Journal of Neurosurgery*, 1984, *61*, 9–16.

Levy, S. *Behavior and cancer*. San Francisco: Jossey-Bass, 1985.

Levy, S.M. The process of death and dying: Behavioral and social factors. In T.G. Burish & L.A. Bradley (Eds.), *Coping with chronic disease: Research and applications*. New York: Academic Press, 1983.

Levy, S.M., Herberman, R.B., Maluish, A.M., Schlien, B., & Lippman, M. Prognostic risk assessment in primary breast cancer by behavioral and immunological parameters. *Health Psychology*, 1985, *4*, 99–113.

Lewis, D.O., Comite, F., Mallouh, C., Zadunaisky, L., Hutchinson-Williams, K., Cherksey, B.D., & Yeager, C. Bipolar mood disorder and endometriosis: Preliminary findings. *American Journal of Psychiatry*, 1987, *144*(12), 1588–1590.

Li, F.P., Cassady, J.P., & Jaffe, N. Risk of second tumors in survivors of childhood cancer. *Cancer*, 1975, *35*, 1230–1235.

Links, P.S., & Kaplan, K.H. The spouses of your heart attack patients: Ways of helping with their emotional response. *Canadian Family Physician*, 1980, *26*, 425, 427–428.

Livesley, W.J. Factors associated with psychiatric symptoms in patients undergoing chronic hemodialysis. *Canadian Journal of Psychiatry*, 1981, *26*(8), 562–566.

Livnat, S., & Felten, D.J. Disease as a reflection of the psyche (letter). *New England Journal of Medicine*, 1985, *313*(21), 1357.

Livneh, H. Death attitudes and their relationship to perceptions of physically disabled persons. *Journal of Rehabilitation*, 1985, *51*(1), 38–41, 80.

Lord, P., Ritvo, S., & Solnit, A.J. Patients' reactions to the death of the psychoanalyst. *International Journal of Psychoanalysis*, 1978, *59*, 189–197.

Louhivuori, K.A., & Hakama, M. Risk of suicide among cancer patients. *American Journal of Epidemiology*, 1979, *35*, 89–100.

Lowery, B.J., & DuCette, J.P. Disease-related learning and disease control in diabetics as a function of locus of control. *Nursing Research*, 1976, *25*, 358.

Luscomb, R.L., Clum, G.A., & Patsiokas, A.T. Mediating factors in the relationship between life stress and suicide attempting. *Journal of Nervous and Mental Disease*, 1980, *168*, 644–650.

Lyles, J.N., Burish, T.G., Krozely, M.G., & Oldham, R.K. (1982). Efficacy of relaxation training and guided imagery in reducing the adverseness of cancer chemotherapy. *Journal of Consulting and Clinical Psychology*, 1982, *50*, 509–529.

Macgregor, F.C. Psychic trauma of facial disfigurement. *Trial*, January 1984, pp. 90–92.

MacKay, A. Self-poisoning—A complication of epilepsy. *British Journal of Psychiatry*, 1979, *134*, 277–282.

Maguire, G.P., Lee, E.G., Bevington, D.J., Kuchemann, C.S., Crabtree, R.J., & Cornell, C.E. Psychiatric problems in the first year after mastectomy. *British Medical Journal*, 1978, *1*, 963–965.

Maguire, P.H., & Asken, M.J. Psychological problems in family practice: Implications for training. *Journal of Clinical Child Psychology*, 1978, *7*, 13–16.

Maguire, P., Tait, A., Brooke, M., Thomas, C., & Sellwood, R. Effects of counseling on the psychiatric morbidity associated with mastectomy. *British Medical Journal*, 1980, *281*, 1454–1456.

Major, R.H. *Classic descriptions of disease*. Springfield, IL: Charles C Thomas, 1965, pp. 240–242.

Margolis, G.J., Carabell, S.C., & Goodman, R.L. Psychological aspects of primary radiation therapy for breast carcinoma. *American Journal of Clinical Oncology*, 1983, *6*(5), 533–538.

Marshak, L. Group therapy with adolescents. In M. Seligman (Ed.), *Group psychotherapy and counseling with special populations*. Baltimore: University Park Press, 1982.

Marshall, J.R., Burnett, W., & Brasure, J. On precipitating factors: Cancer as a cause of suicide. *Suicide and Life-Threatening Behavior*, 1983, *13*(1), 15–17.

Matthews, W., & Barabas, G. Suicide and epilepsy: A review of the literature. *Psychosomatics*, 1981, *22*, 515–524.

Mauss-Clum, N., & Ryan, M. Brain injury and the family. *Journal of Neurosurgical Nursing*, 1981, *4*, 165–169.

Max, G. Psychotherapy with epileptic patients. In R. Canger, F. Aneleri, & J.K. Penry (Eds.), *Advances in epileptology: XIth Epilepsy International Symposium*. New York: Raven Press, 1980.

Mayou, R., Foster, A., & Williamson, B. The psychological and social effects of myocardial infarction on wives. *British Medical Journal*, 1978, *1*, 699–701.

McGovern, H. Comment on Robert's criticism of biofeedback. *American Psychologist*, 1986, *41*, 1007.

McNeil, B., Pauker, S., Sox, H., Jr., & Tversky, A. On the elicitation of preferences for alternative therapies. *New England Journal of Medicine*, 1982, *306*, 1259–1262.

Mechanic, D. Social psychological factors affecting the presentation of bodily complaints. *New England Journal of Medicine*, 1972, *286*, 1132–1139.

Mehta, J., & Krop, H. The effect of myocardial infarction on sexual functioning. *Sexuality and Disability*, 1979, *2*, 115–121.

Menninger, K. *Theory of psychoanalytic technique*. New York: Harper & Row, 1958.

Messerli, M.L., Garamendi, C., & Romano, J. Breast cancer: Information as a technique of crisis intervention. *American Journal of Orthopsychiatry*, 1980, *50*, 728–731.

Meyerowitz, B.E., Heinrich, R.L., & Shag, C.C., A competency-based approach to coping with cancer. In T.G. Burish & L.A. Bradley (Eds.), *Coping with chronic disease: Research and applications*. New York: Academic Press, 1983.

Meyerowitz, B.E., Sparks, F.C., & Spears, I.K. Adjuvant chemotherapy for breast carcinoma: Psychosocial implications. *Cancer*, 1979, *43*, 1613–1618.

Miller, S.M. Predictability and human stress: Towards a clarification of evidence and theory. In L. Berkowitz (Ed.), *Advances in experimental social psychology* (Vol. 14). New York: Academic Press, 1981.

Miller, S.M., & Mangan, C.E. Interacting effects of information and coping style in adapting to gynecologic stress: Should the doctor tell all? *Journal of Personality and Social Psychology*, 1983, *45*(1), 223–236.

Mine, J.F., Golden, J.S., & Fibus, L. Sexual dysfunction in renal failure: A survey of chronic hemodialysis patients. *International Journal of Psychiatry in Medicine*, 1978, *8*, 335–346.

Minuchin, S. *Families and family therapy*. Cambridge, MA: Harvard University Press, 1974.

Minuchin, S., Baker, L., Rosman, B.L., Liebman, R., Milman, L., & Todd, T.C. A conceptual model of psychosomatic illness in children: Family organization and family therapy. *Archives of General Psychiatry*, 1975, *32*, 1031–1038.

Minuchin, S., Rosman, B.L., & Baker, L. *Psychosomatic families: Anorexia nervosa in context*. Cambridge, MA: Harvard University Press, 1978.

Mitchell, G.W., & Glicksman, A.S. Cancer patients: Knowledge and attitudes. *Cancer*, 1977, *40*, 61–66.

Moore, J.E., & Chaney, E.F. Outpatient group treatment of chronic pain: Effects of spouse involvement. *Journal of Consulting and Clinical Psychology*, 1985, *53*(3), 326–334.

Moran, M.G. Psychiatric aspects of tuberculosis. *Advances in Psychosomatic Medicine*, 1985, *14*, 109–118.

Morley, G., Lindenaver, S.M., & Youngs, D. Vaginal reconstruction following pelvic exenteration: Surgical and psychological considerations. *American Journal of Obstetrics and Gynecology*, 1973, *114*, 162–171.

Morrison, M.M., & Ursprung, A.W. Children's attitudes toward people with disabilities: A review of the literature. *Journal of Rehabilitation*, 1987, *53*(1), 45–48.

Morrow, G.R. Prevalence and correlates of anticipatory nausea and vomiting in chemotherapy patients. *Journal of the National Cancer Institute*, 1982, *68*, 585–588.

Morrow, G., Gootnick, B., & Schmale, A. A simple technique for increasing cancer patients' knowledge of informed consent to treatment. *Cancer*, 1978, *42*, 793–799.

Morrow, G.R., & Morrell, C. Behavior treatment for anticipatory nausea and vomiting induced by cancer chemotherapy. *New England Journal of Medicine*, 1982, *307*, 1476–1480.

Mumford, E., Schlesinger, H.J., & Glass, G.V. The effects of psychological intervention on recovery from surgery and heart attacks: An analysis of the literature. *American Journal of Public Health*, 1982, *72*, 141–151.

Nahmias, A.J., Naib, S.M., & Josey, W.E. Epidemiological studies relating genital herpetic infection to cervical carcinoma. *Cancer Research*, 1974, *34*, 1111–1117.

Nakane, Y., Okuma, T., Takahashi, R., Sato, Y., Wada, T., Sato, T., Fukushima, Y., Kumashiro, H., Ono, T., Takahashi, T., Aoki, Y., Kazamatsuri, H., Inami, M., Komai, S., Seino, M., Miyakoshi, M., Tanimura, T., Hazama, H., Kawahara, R., Otsuki, S., Hosokawa, K., Inanaga, K., Nakazawa, Y., & Yamamoto, K. Multi-institutional study on the teratogenicity and fetal toxicity of antiepileptic drugs: A report of a collaborative study group in Japan. *Epilepsia*, 1980, *21*, 663–680.

National Cancer Institute, National Institutes of Health, U.S. Department of Health and Human Services. *Coping with cancer: A resource for the health professional* (NIH Publication No. 80-2080). Washington, DC: U.S. Government Printing Office, 1980.

National Cancer Institute. *Cancer of the prostate: Research report* (NIH Publication No. 81-528). Washington, DC: Author, May 1981.

National Cancer Institute. Surveillance Epidemiology and End Results Program (SEER) cancer patient survival statistics. *Update: Annual Cancer Statistics Review*, 1984, November 26, 1–8.

National Hemlock Society. Most Americans think there should be a legal right-to-die. *Hemlock Quarterly*, 1986, *24*, 1–3.

National Hemlock Society. 60% support in polls. *Hemlock Quarterly*, 1987, *28*, 1.

National Institute of Handicapped Research. *The late effects of poliomyelitis* (Office of Special Education and Rehabilitative Services, Rehabilitation Brief ISSN: 0732-2623, *9*(9)). Falls Church, VA: PSI International, 1986.

Nerenz, D.R., & Leventhal, H. Self-regulation theory in chronic illness. In T.G. Burish & L.A. Bradley (Eds.), *Coping with chronic disease: Research and applications.* New York: Academic Press, 1983.

Nesse, R.M., Carli, T., Curtis, G.C., & Kleinman, P.D. Pretreatment nausea in cancer chemotherapy: A conditioned response? *Psychosomatic Medicine*, 1980, *42*, 33–36.

Norris, P.A. On the status of biofeedback and clinical practice. *American Psychologist*, 1986, *41*, 1009–1010.

Novack, D.H., Plumer, R., Smith, R.I., Octhill, H., Morrow, G.R., & Bennett, J.M. Changes in physicians' attitudes toward telling the cancer patient. *Journal of the American Medical Association*, 1979, *241*, 897–900.

Nunes, E.V., Frank, K.A., & Kornfeld, D. Psychologic treatment for the Type A behavior pattern and for coronary heart disease: A meta-analysis of the literature. *Psychosomatic Medicine*, 1987, *48*(2), 159–171.

Oehler-Giarratana, J., & Fitzgerald, R. Group therapy with blind diabetics. *Archives of General Psychiatry*, 1980, *37*, 463–467.

Oken, D. What to tell cancer patients: A study of medical attitudes. *Journal of the American Medical Association*, 1961, *175*, 1120–1128.

Olafsdottir, M., Sjoden, P., & Westling, B. Prevalence and prediction of chemotherapy-related anxiety, nausea and vomiting in cancer patients. *Behaviour Research and Therapy*, 1986, *24*(1), 59–66.

Oradei, D.M., & Waite, N.S. Group psychotherapy with stroke patients during the immediate recovery phase. *American Journal of Orthopsychiatry*, 1974, *44*, 386–395.

Parker, L.H., & Baer, G.R. Neurological and neuromuscular disorders. In K.A. Holroyd & T.L. Creer (Eds.), *Self-management of chronic disease*. New York: Academic Press, 1986.

Pattison, F.M., Rhohdes, R.J., & Dudley, D.L. Response to group treatment in patients with severe chronic lung disease. *International Journal of Group Psychotherapy*, 1971, *21*, 214.

Pavlidis, N., & Chirigos, M. Stress induced impairment of macrophage tumoricidal function. *Psychosomatic Medicine*, 1980, *42*, 47–54.

Peck, A., & Boland, J. Emotional reactions to radiation treatment. *Cancer*, 1977, *40*, 180–184.

Perry, D.C., & Apostal, R.A. Modifying attitudes of business leaders toward disabled persons. *Journal of Rehabilitation*, 1986, *52*(4), 35–38.

Persky, V.W., Kempthorne-Rawson, J., & Shekelle, R.B. Personality and risk of cancer: 20-year follow-up of the Western Electric Study. *Psychosomatic Medicine*, 1987, 435–449.

Piscor, B.K., & Paleos, S. The group way to banish after-stroke blues. *American Journal of Nursing*, 1968, *68*, 1500–1503.

Plumb, M., & Holland, J. Comparative studies of psychological function in patients with advanced cancer II. Interviewer-rated current and past psychological symptoms. *Psychosomatic Medicine*, 1981, *43*(3), 243–254.

Podolsky, S. Diagnosis and treatment of sexual dysfunction in the male diabetic. *Medical Clinics of North America*, 1982, *66*, 1389–1396.

Polivy, J. Psychological effects of mastectomy on a woman's feminine self-concept. *Journal of Nervous and Mental Disease*, 1977, *164*, 77–87.

Poulton, T.J., & Powell-Butdorf, M.B. Death in the ICU: Does the patient predict his own demise? *Critical Care Medicine*, 1986, *14*(7), 614–616.

Pow, J.M. The role of psychological influences in rheumatoid arthritis. *Journal of Psychosomatic Research*, 1987, *31*(2), 223–229.

Power, P.W., & Del Orto, A.E. Impact of disability illness on the child. In P.W. Power & A.E. Del Orto (Eds.), *Role of the family in the rehabilitation of the physically disabled*. Baltimore: University Park Press, 1980, pp. 111–116.

Preston, C. Behavior modification: A therapeutic approach to aging and dying. *Postgraduate Medicine*, 1973, *54*, 67–68.

Pritchard, P.B., Lombroso, C.T., & McIntyre, M. Psychological complications of temporal lobe epilepsy. *Neurology*, 1980, *30*, 227–232.

Procci, W., Hoffman, K., & Chatterjee, S.A. Sexual functioning of renal transplant patients. *Journal of Nervous and Mental Disease*, 1978, *166*, 402–407.

Prokop, C.K., & Bradley, L.A. Methodological issues in medical psychology and behavioral medicine research. In C.K. Prokop & L.A. Bradley (Eds)., *Medical psychology: Contributions to behavioral medicine*. New York: Academic Press, 1981.

Prudhomme, C. Epilepsy and suicide. *Journal of Nervous and Mental Disease*, 1941, *94*, 722–731.

Rabin, C., Amir, S., Nardi, R., & Ovadia, B. Compliance and control issues in group training for diabetics. *Health and Social Work*, 1986, *11*(2), 141–151.

Rabkin, J.B., & Struening, E.L. Life experiences, stress and illness. *Science*, 1976, *194*, 1013–1020.

Radovsky, S.S. Bearing the news. *New England Journal of Medicine*, 1985, *313*(9), 586–588.

Ragland, D.R., & Brand, R.J. Type A behavior and mortality from coronary heart disease. *New England Journal of Medicine*, 1988, *318*(2), 65–69.

Rahe, R.H., O'Neil, T., Hagan, A., & Arthur, R.J. Brief group therapy following myocardial infarction: Eighteen month follow-up of a controlled trial. *International Journal of Psychiatry in Medicine*, 1975, *6*, 349–358.

Rahe, R.H., Ward, H.W., & Hayes, V. Brief group therapy in myocardial infarction rehabilitation: Three to four-year follow-up of a controlled trial. *Psychosomatic Medicine*, 1979, *41*, 229–242.

Ramsey, P. *The patient as person*. New Haven: Yale University Press, 1972.

Rando, T.A. An investigation of grief and adaptation in parents whose children have died from cancer. *Journal of Pediatric Psychology*, 1983, *8*, 3–20.

Rasmussen, J.E. Minor surgical procedures in children. *Journal of Dermatologic Surgery and Oncology*, 1982, *8*, 706–707.

Redd, W.H., Andersen, G.V., & Minagawa, R.Y. Hypnotic control of anticipatory emesis in patients receiving cancer chemotherapy. *Journal of Consulting and Clinical Psychology*, 1982, *50*, 14–19.

Resuming sex after heart surgery. *Health Letter* (NYU Medical Center), 1987, *1*(9), 3.

Review Panel on Coronary-Prone Behaviour and Coronary Heart Disease. Coronary-prone behavior and coronary heart disease: A critical review. *Circulation*, 1981, *63*, 1199–1215.

Ringler, K.E. *Processes of coping with cancer chemotherapy*. Unpublished doctoral dissertation, University of Wisconsin-Madison, 1981.

Roberts, A.H. Biofeedback: Research, training, and clinical roles. *American Psychologist*, 1985, *40*, 938–941.

Roberts, A.H. Biofeedback, science, and training. *American Psychologist*, 1986, *41*, 1010.

Rodin, G., & Voshart, K. Depression in the medically ill: An overview. *American Journal of Psychiatry*, 1986, *143*(6), 696–705.

Rodin, G.M., Chmara, J., Ennis, J., Fenton, S., Locking, H., & Steinhouse, K. Stopping life-sustaining medical treatment: Psychiatric considerations in the termination of renal dialysis. *Canadian Journal of Psychiatry*, 1981, *26*(8), 540–544.

Roeske, N.C.A. Hysterectomy and other gynecological surgeries: A psychological view. In M.F. Notman & C.C. Nadelson (Eds.), *The woman patient: Medical and psychological interfaces*. New York: Plenum Press, 1978.

Rogentine, G.N., van Kammen, D.P., Fox, B.H., Docherty, J.P.., Rosenblatt, J.E., Boyd, S.C., & Bunney, W.E. Psychological factors in the prognosis of malignant melanoma: A prospective study. *Psychosomatic Medicine*, 1979, *41*, 647–655.

Rogers, M., & Reich, P. Psychological intervention with surgical patients: Evaluation outcome. *Advances in Psychosomatic Medicine*, 1986, *15*, 23–50.

Roll, M., & Theorell, T. Acute chest pain without obvious organic cause before 40—Personality and recent life events. *Journal of Psychosomatic Research*, 1987, *31*(2), 215–221.

Roosevelt Warm Springs Institute for Rehabilitation, Warm Springs, Georgia. *Polio News*, 1982, *1*(2), 2–5.

Roosevelt Warm Springs Institute for Rehabilitation, Warm Springs, Georgia. *Polio News*, 1983, *1*(1), 2–4.

Rosen, J.C., & Wiens, A.N. Changes in medical problems and use of medical services following psychological intervention. *American Psychologist*, 1979, *34*(5), 420–431.

Rosenman, R.H. The impact of anxiety on the cardiovascular system. *Psychosomatics*, 1985, *26*(11), 6–15.

Rosenman, R.H., Brand, R.J., Shaltz, R.L., & Friedman, M. Multivariate prediction of coronary heart disease during 8.5 year follow-up in the Western Collaborative Group Study. *American Journal of Cardiology*, 1976, *37*, 903–910.

Roth, D.L., & Holmes, D.S.Influence of aerobic exercise training and relaxation training on physical and psychologic health following stressful life events. *Psychosomatic Medicine*, 1987, *49*, 355–365.

Roth, S., & Cohen, L.J. Approach, avoidance, and coping with stress. *American Psychologist*, 1986, *41*(7), 813–819.

Rotman, M. Rogow, L., DeLeon, G., & Heskel, N. Supportive therapy in radiation oncology. *Cancer*, 1977, *39*, 744–750.

Rotter, J.B. Generalized expectancies for internal versus external control of reinforcement. *Psychological Monographs*, 1966, *80*(1, 609), 1–28.

Ruberman, W., Weinblatt, E., Goldberg, J.D., & Chaudhary, B.S., Psychosocial influences on mortality after myocardial infarction. *New England Journal of Medicine*, 1984, *311*(9), 552–559.

Rundell, J.R., Wise, M.G., & Ursano, R.J. Three cases of AIDS-related psychiatric disorders. *American Journal of Psychiatry*, 1986, *143*(6), 777–778.

Ryan, C.M., & Morrow, L.A. Self-esteem in diabetic adolescents: Relationship between age at onset and gender. *Journal of Consulting and Clinical Psychology*, 1986, *54*(5), 730–731.

Sawyer, J.D., Adams, K.M., Conway, W.L., Reeves, J., & Kvale, P.A. Suicide in cases of chronic obstructive pulmonary disease. *Journal of Psychiatric Treatment and Evaluation*, 1983, *5*, 281–283.

Schain, W.S. Sexual problems of patients with cancer. In S. Hellman, V. DiVita, Jr., & S.A. Rosenberg (Eds.), *Cancer: Principles and practice of oncology*. Philadelphia: Lippincott, 1982.

Schatzkin, A., Jones, D.Y., Hoover, R.N., Taylor, P.R., Brinton, L.A., Ziegler, R.G., Harvey, E.B., Carter, C.L., Licitra, L.M., Dufour, M.C., & Larson, D.B. Alcohol consumption and breast cancer in the epidemiologic follow-up study of the first national health and nutrition examination survey. *New England Journal of Medicine*, 1987, *316*(19), 1169–1173.

Schneiderman, N., & Tapp, J.T. *Behavioral medicine: A biopsychological approach*. Hillsdale, NJ: Erlbaum, 1983.

Schoenfeld, M., Myers, R.H., Cupples, L.A., Berkman, B., Sax, D.S., & Clark, E. Increased rate of suicide among patients with Huntington's disease. *Journal of Neurology, Neurosurgery, and Psychiatry*, 1984, *47*, 1283–1287.

Schover, L.R., von Eschenbach, A.C., Smith, D.B., & Gonzales, J. Sexual rehabilitation of urologic cancer patients: A practical approach. *Ca: A Cancer Journal for Clinicians*, 1984, *34*, 67–74.

Schroeder, P.S., & Miller, J.K. Qualitative study of locus of control in patients with peripheral vascular disease. In J.F. Miller (Ed.), *Coping with chronic illness: Overcoming powerlessness*, Philadelphia: Davis, 1983, pp. 149–161.

Schuler, R.S. Dealing with the effects of work-related stress. *American Journal of Medical Technology*, 1982, *48*(3), 177–182.

Schwab, J.J. Psychiatric illness in medical patients: Why it goes undiagnosed. *Psychosomatics*, 1982, *23*, 225–229.

Schwartz, M., & Cahill, R. Psychopathology associated with myasthenia gravis and its treatment in psychotherapeutically oriented group counseling. *Journal of Chronic Diseases*, 1971, *24*, 543.

Scurry, M.T., & Levin, E.M. Psychosocial factors related to the incidence of cancer. *International Journal of Psychiatry in Medicine*, 1978–1979, *9*(2), 159–177.

Seeman, M., & Evans, J. Alienation and learning in a hospital setting. *American Sociological Review*, 1962, *27*, 772–782.

Seeman, T.E., & Syme, S.L. Social networks and coronary artery disease: A comparison of the structure and function of social relations as predictors of disease. *Psychosomatic Medicine*, 1987, *49*, 341–354.

Seigel, L.J., & Longo, D.L. The control of chemotherapy-induced emesis. *Annals of Internal Medicine*, 1981, *95*, 359.

Shapiro, J. Assessment of family coping with illness. *Psychosomatics*, 1986, *27*(4), 262–271.

Shapiro, J., & Tittle, K. Individual and family correlates among poor, Spanish-speaking women and their attitudes and responses to children and adults with disabilities. *Journal of Rehabilitation*, 1986, *52*(4), 61–65.

Shekelle, R.B., Hulley, S.B., Neaton, J.D., Billings, J.H., Borhani, N.O., Gerace, T.A., Jacobs, D.R., Lasser, N.L., Mittlemark, M.B., & Stamler, J., for the Multiple Risk Factor Intervention Trial Research Group. The MRFIT behavior pattern study, II. Type A behavior and incidence of coronary heart disease. *American Journal of Epidemiology*, 1985, *122*, 559–570.

Sheldon, A., Ryser, C.P., & Krant, M.J. An integrated family oriented cancer care program. *Journal of Chronic Disease*, 1970, *22*, 743–755.

Shipley, R.H., Butt, J.H., Horowitz, E.A., & Farbry, J.E. Preparation for a stressful medical procedure: Effect of amount of stimulus pre-exposure and coping style. *Journal of Consulting and Clinical Psychology*, 1978, *46*, 499–507.

Shneidman, E.S. Some aspects of psychotherapy with dying persons. In C.A. Garfield (Ed.), *Psychosocial care of the dying patient*. New York: McGraw-Hill, 1978.

Shontz, F.C. The personal meaning of illness. *Advances in Psychosomatic Medicine*, 1972, *8*, 63–85.

Shontz, F.C. *The psychological aspects of physical illness and disability*. New York: McGraw-Hill, 1975.

Shwed, H.J. When a psychiatrist dies. *Journal of Nervous and Mental Disease*, 1980, *168*(5), 275–278.

Siegel, K., & Tuckel, P. Rational suicide and the terminally ill cancer patient. *Omega*, 1984–1985, *15*(3), 263–269.

Siegman, A.W., Dembroski, T.M., & Ringel, N. Components of hostility and the severity of coronary artery disease. *Psychosomatic Medicine*, 1987, *49*(2), 127–134.

Silberfarb, P.M., Mauer, L.H., & Crouthamel, C.S. Psychosocial aspects of neoplastic disease, I: Functional status of breast cancer patients during different treatment regimens. *American Journal of Psychiatry*, 1980, *137*, 450–455.

Siller, F. Reactions to physical disability. *Rehabilitation Counseling Bulletin*, 1963, *7*, 12–16.

Silver, P.S., Auerbach, S.M., Vishniavsky, N., & Kaplowitz, L.G. Psychological factors in recurrent genital herpes infection: Stress, coping style, social support, emotional dysfunction, and symptom recurrence. *Journal of Psychosomatic Research*, 1986, *30*(2), 163–171.

Silverman, S. Psychoanalytic observations on vulnerability to physical disease. *Journal of the American Academy of Psychoanalysis*, 1985, *13*(3), 295–315.

Simonton, O.C., Matthews-Simonton, S., & Creighton, J. *Getting well again: A step by step, self-help guide to overcoming cancer for patients and their families*. Los Angeles: Tarcher, 1978.

Simonton, O.C., Matthews-Simonton, S., & Sparks, T.F. Psychological intervention in the treatment of cancer. *Psychosomatics* 1980, *21*, 226–233.

Singler, J.K. Group work with hospitalized stroke patients. *Social Casework*, 1975, *56*, 348–354.

Singler, J.K. The use of groups with stroke patients. In M. Seligman (Ed.), *Group counselling and group psychotherapy with rehabilitation clients*. Springfield, IL: Thomas, 1977.

Singler, J.K. The stroke group. In M. Seligman (Ed.), *Group psychotherapy and counseling with special populations*. Baltimore: University Park Press, 1981.

Sjodin, I., Svedlund, J., Ottosson, J., & Dotevall, G. Controlled study of psychotherapy in chronic peptic ulcer disease. *Psychosomatics*, 1986, *27*(3), 187–197.

Sjogren, K., & Fugl-Meyer, A.R. Adjustment to life after stroke with special reference to sexual intercourse and leisure. *Journal of Psychosomatic Research*, 1982, *26*, 409–417.

Skeleton, M., & Dominian, J. Psychological stress in wives of patients with myocardial infarction. *British Medical Journal*, 1973, *2*, 101–103.

Sklar, L.S., & Anisman, H. Stress and cancer. *Psychological Bulletin*, 1981, *89*, 369–406.

Sklar, L.S., Bruto, V., & Anisman, H. Adaptation to the tumor-enhancing effects of stress. *Psychosomatic Medicine*, 1981, *43*, 331–342.

Slavin, L., O'Malley, J.E., Koocher, G.P., & Foster, D.J. Communication of the cancer diagnosis to pediatric patients: Impact on long-term adjustment. *American Journal of Psychiatry*, 1981, *139*, 179–183.

Smith, J.C. Meditation, biofeedback, and the relaxation controversy: A cognitive-behavior perspective. *American Psychologist*, 1986, *41*, 1007–1009.

Smith, M.L., Glass, G.V., & Miller, T.S. *The benefit of psychotherapy*. Baltimore: Johns Hopkins University Press, 1980.

Sobel, H. Toward a behavioral thanatology in clinical care. In H. Sobel (Ed.), *Behavioral therapy in terminal care: A humanistic approach.* Cambridge, MA: Ballinger, 1981.

Soloff, P.H. The liaison psychiatrist in cardiovascular rehabilitation: An overview. *International Journal of Psychiatry in Medicine, 1977–1978, 8,* 393–403.

Solomon, G.F. The emerging field of psychoneuroimmunology. *Advances: Journal of the Institute for the Advancement of Health, 1985, 2,* 6–19.

Sontag, S. *Illness as metaphor.* New York: Vintage, 1979.

Spiegel, D. Psychological support for women with metastatic carcinoma. *Psychosomatics, 1979, 20,* 780–785.

Spiegel, D., Bloom, J., & Yalom, I. Group support for patients with metastatic cancer. *Archives of General Psychiatry, 1981, 20,* 780–784.

Spinetta, J.J., Swarmer, J.A., & Sheposh, J.P. Effective parental coping following the death of a child from cancer. *Journal of Pediatric Psychology, 1981, 6,* 251–263.

Steering Committee on the Physician's Health Study Research Group. Preliminary Report: Findings from the aspirin component of the on-going Physician's Health Study. *New England Journal of Medicine, 1988, 318*(4), 262–264.

Stern, M.J., & Pascale, L. Psychosocial adaptation post myocardial infarction: The spouse's dilemma. *Journal of Psychosomatic Research, 1979, 23,* 83–87.

Stevens, J.R. Complex partial seizures (psychomotor epilepsy): Interictal manifestations. In J.R. Penry & D.D. Daly (Eds.), *Complex partial seizures.* New York: Raven Press, 1975.

Stevens, J.R. Biologic background of psychoses in epilepsy. In R. Canger, F. Angeleri, & J.K. Penry (Eds.), *Advances in epileptology: XIth Epilepsy International Symposium.* New York: Raven Press, 1980.

Stone, R. Employing the recovered cancer patient. *Cancer, 1975, 36,* 285–286.

Stoudemire, A. Psychosomatic theory and pulmonary disease: Asthma as a paradigm for the biopsychosocial approach. *Advances in Psychosomatic Medicine, 1985, 14,* 1–15.

Streltzer, J. Psychiatric aspects of oncology: A review of recent research. *Hospital and Community Psychiatry, 1983, 34*(8), 716–723.

Studies show there's room for improvement. *The Internist* (American Society of Internal Medicine), August 1986, p. 9.

Sullivan, H.S. Conceptions of modern psychiatry. Reprinted from *Psychiatry, 1940, 3,* 1–117; 1945, 8, 177–205. Washington, DC: William Alanson White Psychiatric Foundation, 1947.

Tapp, J.T. Health psychology; An evolving discipline for psychologists. *Psychotherapy in Private Practice, 1984, 2*(1), 49–64.

Tattersall, R.B., McCulloch, D.K., & Aveline, M. Group therapy in the treatment of diabetes. *Diabetes Care, 1985, 8,* 180–188.

Taylor, C.M., & Crisler, J.R. Concerns of persons with cancer as perceived by cancer patients, physicians, and rehabilitation counselors. *Journal of Rehabilitation, 1988, 54*(1), 23–27.

Taylor, D.C. Factors influencing the occurrence of schizophrenic-like psychosis in patients with temporal lobe epilepsy. *Psychological Medicine, 1975, 5,* 249–254.

Taylor, S. Adjustment to threatening events: A theory of cognitive adaptation. *American Psychologist, 1983, 38,* 1161–1173.

Taylor, S.E., Falke, R.L., Shoptaw, S.J., & Lichtman, R.R. Social support, support groups, and the cancer patient. *Journal of Consulting and Clinical Psychology, 1986, 54*(5), 608–615.

Taylor, S.E., Lichtman, R.R., & Wood, J.V. Attributions, beliefs about control and adjustment to breast cancer. *Journal of Personality and Social Psychology, 1984, 46,* 489–502.

Tessler, R., Mechanic, D., & Dimond, M. The effect of psychological distress on physician utilization: A prospective study. *Journal of Health and Social Behavior, 1976, 17,* 353–364.

Thomas, C., Madden, F., & Jehu, D. Psychological effects of stomas—I. Psychosocial morbidity one year after surgery. *Journal of Psychosomatic Research, 1987, 31*(3), 311–316. (a)

Thomas, C., Madden F., & Jehu, D. Psychological effects of stomas—II Factors influencing outcome. *Journal of Psychosomatic Research, 1987, 31*(3), 317–323. (b)

Thomas, J. Problems in a study of the sexual response of women with cancer: Comment on Andersen and Jochimsen. *Journal of Consulting and Clinical Psychology*, 1987, *55*(1), 120–121.

Thompson, S.C. A complex response to simple question: Will it hurt less if I can control it? *Psychological Bulletin*, 1981, *90*, 89–101.

Thompson, W.L, & Thompson, T.L, II. Psychiatric aspects of asthma in adults. *Advances in Psychosomatic Medicine*, 1985, *14*, 33–47.

Trillin, A.S. Of dragons and garden peas: A cancer patient talks to doctors. *New England Journal of Medicine*, 1981, *304*, 699–701.

Tulkin, S.R., & Frank, G.W. The changing role of psychologists in health maintenance organizations. *American Psychologist*, 1985, *40*(10), 1125–1130.

Turk, D.C., & Rudy, T.E. Assessment of cognitive factors in chronic pain: A worthwhile enterprise? *Journal of Counseling and Clinical Psychology*, 1986, *54*(6), 760–768.

Turk, J. Impact of cystic fibrosis on family functioning. *Pediatrics*, 1964, *34*, 67–71.

Turkington, C. Disfigured need help for inner wounds. *American Psychological Association Monitor*, July 1984, pp. 6–7.

Turns, D., & Sands, R.G. Psychological problems of patients with head and neck cancer. *Journal of Prosthetic Dentistry*, 1978, *39*(1), 68–73.

Tversky, A., & Kahneman, D. The framing of decisions and the psychology of choice. *Science*, 1981, *211*, 452–458.

Tyler, A., Harper, P.S., Davies, K., & Newcome, R.G. Family break-down and stress in Huntington's chorea. *Journal of Biosocial Science*, 1983, *15*, 127–138.

Udelman, H.D., & Udelman, D.L. Group therapy with rheumatoid arthritic patients. *American Journal of Psychotherapy*, 1978, *32*, 288-299.

U.S. Bureau of the Census. *Statistical abstracts of the United States* (105th ed.). Washington, DC: U.S. Government Printing Office, 1985.

Vachon, M.L.S., Lyall, W.A.L., Rogers, J., Cochrane, J., & Freeman, S.J.J. The effectiveness of psychosocial support during post-surgical treatment of breast cancer. *International Journal of Psychiatry in Medicine*, 1981–1982, *11*(4), 365–372.

Viney, L.L. Expression of positive emotion by people who are physically ill: Is it evidence of defending or coping? *Journal of Psychosomatic Research*, 1986, *30*(1), 27–34.

Viney, L.L., & Westbrook, M.T. Psychological reactions to chronic illness-related disability as a function of its severity and type. *Journal of Psychosomatic Research*, 1981, *25*(6), 513–523.

Waitzkin, H. Doctor–patient communication: Clinical implications of social scientific research. *Journal of the American Medical Association*, 1984, *252*(17), 2441–2446.

Waitzkin, H. Information giving in medical care. *Journal of Health and Social Behavior*, 1985, *26*(June), 81–101.

Waitzkin, H. Research on doctor–patient communication. *The Internist* (American Society of Internal Medicine), August 1986, pp. 7–10.

Walker, L.A. What comforts AIDS families? *The New York Times Magazine*, June 21, 1987, pp. 16–22, 63, 78.

Wallace, R.K. Physiological effects of transcendental meditation. *Science*, 1970, *167*, 1751–1754.

Washer, G.F., Schroter, G.P.J., Starzl, T.E., & Weil, R. Causes of death after kidney transplantation. *Journal of the American Medical Association*, 1983, *250*(1), 49–54.

Watson, D., & Kendall, P.C. Methodological issues in research on coping with chronic disease. In T.G. Burish & L.A. Bradley (Eds.), *Coping with chronic disease: Research and applications*. New York: Academic Press, 1983.

Weinberger, J.L., & Kantor, M. Possible sequelae of trauma and somatic disorder in early life. *International Journal of Psychiatry in Medicine*, 1976–1977, *7*, 334–350.

Weiner, H. *Psychobiology and human disease*. New York: Elsevier, 1977.

Weinman, B. Membership retention in group therapy among adolescents who are physically disabled. *Journal of Rehabilitation*, 1987, *53*(2), 52–55.

Weisman, A.D. Misgivings and misconceptions in the psychiatric care of terminal ill patients. In C.A. Garfield (Ed.), *Psychosocial care of the dying patient*. New York: McGraw-Hill, 1978.

Weisman, A., & Hackett, T. The dying patient in special treatment situations. Des Plaines, IL: Forest Hospital Publication, *1*, 1962. (C.A. Garfield (Ed.), *Psychosocial care of the dying patient*. New York: McGraw-Hill, 1978.)

Weisman, A.D., & Worden, J.W. Risk rescue rating in suicide assessment. *Archives of General Psychiatry*, 1972, *26*, 553–560.

Weisman, A.D., & Worden, J.W. *Coping and vulnerability in cancer patients: A research report.* Cambridge, MA: Authors, 1977.

Weisman, A.D., Worden, J.W., & Sobel, H.J. *Psychosocial screening and intervention with cancer patients.* Cambridge, MA: Authors, 1980.

Wellisch, D.K., Jamison, K.R., & Pasnau, R.O. Psychosocial aspects of mastectomy, II: The man's perspective. *American Journal of Psychiatry*, 1978, *135*, 443–546.

Wheatley, G., Cunnick, W., Wright, B., & van Keuren, D. The employment of persons with a history of treatment of cancer. *Cancer*, 1974, *33*, 441–445.

White, L., & Tursky, B. Commentary on Roberts. *American Psychologist*, 1986, *41*, 1005–1007.

Whitehead, V.M. Cancer treatment needs better antiemetics. *New England Journal of Medicine*, 1975, *293*, 199–200.

Whitfield, C.L. Co-alcoholism: Recognizing a treatable illness. *Family and Community Health*, 1984, *7*(2), 16–27.

Wilkinson, G. The influence of psychiatric, psychological and social factors on the control of insulin-dependent diabetes mellitus. *Journal of Psychosomatic Research*, 1987, *31*(3), 277–286.

Willett, W.C., Stampfer, M.J., Golditz, G.A., Rosner, B.A., Hennekens, C.H., & Speizer, F.E. Moderate alcohol consumption and the risk of breast cancer. *New England Journal of Medicine*, 1987, *316*(19), 1174–1180.

Williams, J.M., & Stout, J.K. The effect of high and low assertiveness on locus of control and health problems. *Journal of Psychology*, 1985, *119*(2), 169–173.

Williams, K.R., & Stensaas, J. *So you're having an operation: A step by step guide to controlling your hospital stay.* Cliffside, NJ: Prentice-Hall, 1985.

Williams, R.B., Benson, H., & Follick, M.J. Disease as a reflection of the psyche (letter). *New England Journal of Medicine*, 1985, *313*(21), 1356–1357.

Williams, R.B., Haney, T.L., Lee, K.L., Kong, Y., Blumenthal, J.A., & Whalen, R.E. Type A behavior, hostility, and coronary atherosclerosis. *Psychosomatic Medicine*, 1980, *42*(6), 539–549.

Wise, T.N. Sexual dysfunction in the medically ill. *Psychosomatics*, 1983, *24*(9), 787–805.

Wolpe, J. *Practice of behavior therapy* (2nd ed.). New York: Pergamon Press, 1974.

Wolpe, J. Behavior therapy for psychosomatic disorders. *Psychosomatics*, 1980, *21*, 279–285.

Woodburne, C. A survey of adjustment of chronic renal failure and intermittent hemodialysis with particular attention to sexual adjustment. *Nursing*, University of Wisconsin, 1973. (C.A. Garfield (Ed.), *Psychosocial care of the dying patient*. New York: McGraw-Hill, 1978, p. 322.)

Worden, J.W., & Sobel, H.J. Ego strength and psychosocial adaptation to cancer. *Psychosomatic Medicine*, 1978, *40*, 585–592.

Worden, J.W., & Weisman, A.D. Psychosocial components of lagtime in cancer diagnosis. *Journal of Psychosomatic Research*, 1975, *19*, 69–79.

Wright, L. The Type A behavior pattern and coronary artery disease: Quest for the active ingredients and the elusive mechanism. *American Psychologist*, 1988, *43*(1), 2–14.

Yalom, I.D., & Grooves, C. Group therapy with the terminally ill. *American Journal of Psychiatry*, 1977, *134*, 396–400.

Yates, J.W., Chalmer, B.J., St. James, P., Follansbee, M., & McKegney, F.P. Religion in patients with advanced cancer. *Medical and Pediatric Oncology*, 1981, 121–128.

Ziarnik, J.P., Freeman, C.W., Sherrard, D.J., & Calsyn, D.A. Psychological correlates of survival on renal dialysis. *Journal of Nervous and Mental Disease*, 1977, *164*, 210–213.

Ziegler, E.A. Spouses of persons who are brain injured: Overlooked victims. *Journal of Reha-bilitation*, 1987, 5(1), 50–53.
Ziegler, R.G. Impairments of control and competence in epileptic children and their families. *Epilepsia*, 1981, 22, 339–346.

Index